# THE PSYCHOLOGICAL REHABILITATION OF THE AMPUTEE

# The Psychological Rehabilitation Of the Amputee

*By*

LAWRENCE W. FRIEDMANN, M.D.,
F.A.C.A., F.I.C.A.

*Chairman of The Department of Rehabilitation Medicine*
*Nassau County Medical Center*
*East Meadow, New York*
*Professor of Rehabilitation Medicine*
*State University of New York at Stony Brook*
*Stony Brook, New York*
*Associate Professor of Clinical Rehabilitation Medicine*
*New York University*
*New York, New York*
*Former Medical Director*
*Institute for the Crippled and Disabled*
*Rehabilitation and Research Center*
*New York, New York*

CHARLES C THOMAS • PUBLISHER
*Springfield • Illinois • U.S.A.*

*Published and Distributed Throughout the World by*

CHARLES C THOMAS • PUBLISHER
Bannerstone House
301-327 East Lawrence Avenue, Springfield, Illinois, U.S.A.



ISBN 0-398-03707-8

Library of Congress Catalog Card Number 77-23053

*With THOMAS BOOKS careful attention is given to all details of manufacturing and design. It is the Publisher's desire to present books that are satisfactory as to their physical qualities and artistic possibilities and appropriate for their particular use. THOMAS BOOKS will be true to those laws of quality that assure a good name and good will.*

**Library of Congress Cataloging in Publication Data**

Friedmann, Lawrence W
The psychological rehabilitation of the amputee.

Bibliography: p.
Includes index.
1. Amputees—Psychology. 2. Amputees—Rehabilitation. I. Title. [DNLM: 1. Amputees. 2. Amputation. 3. Rehabilitation. WE170 F911p]
RD553.F74 617'.58 77-23053
ISBN 0-398-03707-8

*Printed in the United States of America*
*C-1*

This book is dedicated to my wife, with thanks for the encouragement and help she gives me. Without her, this book could never have been written.

# INTRODUCTION

THE PSYCHOLOGY of the amputee is very complex and fascinating. It is as diverse as human beings. Each person reacts to amputation according to his predisposition. This is modified by his cultural background, training, and resources. The resources are not only psychic but social, vocational, and economic. The pattern of responses varies with the age of the amputee at the time of limb loss. Congenital malformations are responded to in a somewhat different manner than surgical or traumatic limb loss.

The cultural differences are enormous. In certain cultures, limb loss is feared more than death, and patients will willingly die to avoid amputation. This is still true in many of the Arabic countries. The history of amputation is interesting in its own right, but also in how cultures have differed in their attitudes toward the amputee. For that reason, the first chapter of this book on the psychological rehabilitation of the amputee is a chapter on the history of amputation as it relates to societal attitudes to the amputee.

The reactions of society are incorporated into the amputee's self-image. When the greater society responds to the amputee with aversion, the amputee generally incorporates this feeling into his own self-image. This often leads to self-deprecation and self-hate. This in turn may be manifested directly or subtly. In order to compensate for these feelings of lack of self-worth, he may become an "amputee athlete" or a "professional amputee." These individuals excel in one or more activities in order to prove to themselves that they have more worth than they really feel.

This narrow aspect of general psychology may be taken as a paradigm for the reactions to disability.

L.W.F.

# ACKNOWLEDGMENTS

EACH AUTHOR ATTEMPTS to be original, but all of us appreciate how very much we lean on the accumulated wisdom of others, both directly and indirectly.

Many sources of information are acknowledged in this book by direct reference. There are many people whose ideas I have heard and incorporated into my own thinking over the years. Sometimes I have even forgotten from whom I heard a particular piece of information. I hereby wish to thank all of my friends who have helped me in this work, including those who received no direct acknowledgment. I especially wish to thank Doctor Sidney Licht, with whom I originally started to write this book. Unfortunately for me, Doctor Licht retired from all medical responsibilities and left the writing of the book to me. I wish it had been otherwise.

Doctor Allen S. Russek is the friend and teacher who has taught me the most about amputation and amputees. To him I owe a debt that can never be repaid.

I also want to thank my friends, the late Doctor Ernest Spira, Doctor Leonard Bender, Doctor Ernst Marquardt, and the Reverend Harold Wilke.

I owe a large debt to the medical librarian at ICD Rehabilitation and Research Center, Mrs. Helen Stonehill.

The Milbank family and ICD have provided some of the typing in this work and some of the illustrations for subsequent work. The author is most grateful to them and especially to the late S. W. Farnsworth for his constant encouragement and support.

L.W.F.

# CONTENTS

# THE PSYCHOLOGICAL REHABILITATION OF THE AMPUTEE

Chapter I

# A SHORT HISTORY OF AMPUTATION AND ITS PSYCHOLOGY

AMPUTATION is as old as man himself. Its study involves not only the history of medicine, but also archaeology, anthropology, and ethnology. It clarifies what people thought and think of amputees.

The earliest evidence of amputation, about 36,000 years old and found in caves in Spain and France, is a negative imprint of what seem to be deformed hands (Fig. 1). Similar imprints are found from a later date in New Mexico. The widespread practice of self-mutilation was performed to appease the gods and, as such, was a form of "religious rehabilitation."

Congenital deformities and limb absence occurred (Fig. 2), especially in the Arabic countries where first-cousin intermarriage was encouraged (Haj, 1970). All civilizations discouraged the survival of deformed infants, with the sole exception of the

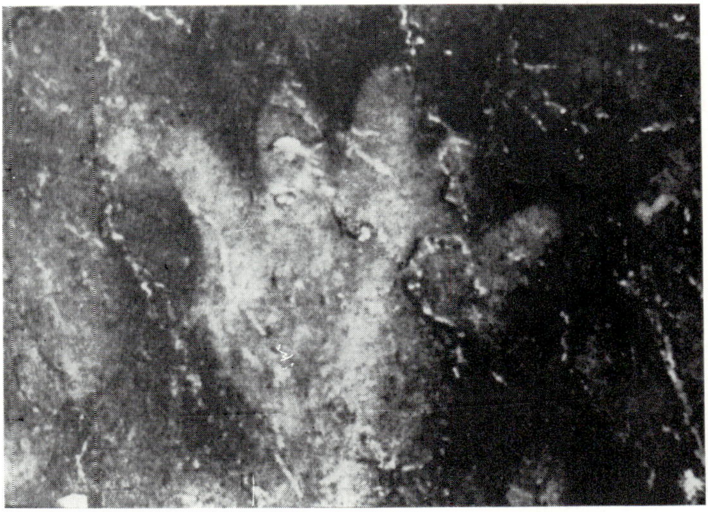

Figure 1. Mutilated-hand negative imprint from Gargas Cave, Spain. Circa 34,000 B.C.E. Courtesy of *Abbottempo*.

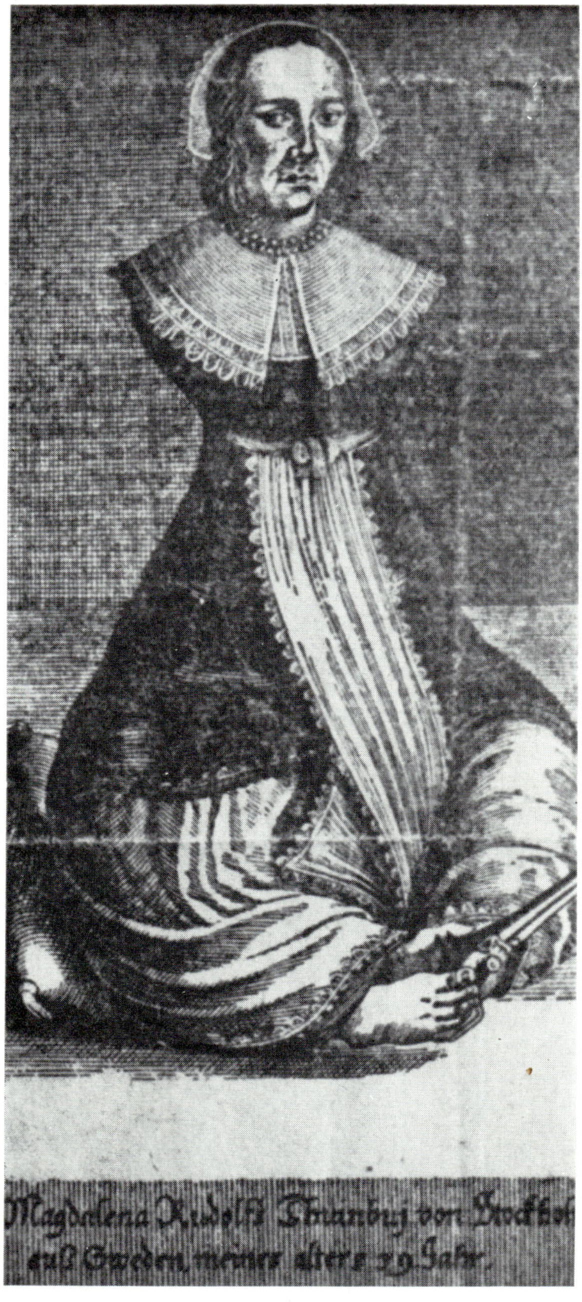

Figure 2. Newspaper illustration, Sweden, 1654, showing woman with bilateral upper amelia firing pistol and doing many other daily activities with her feet. Courtesy of Doctor Ernst Marquardt, Heidelberg, West Germany.

ancient Mexicans. Montezuma II protected the disabled in a special compound for the disabled adjacent to the Royal Zoo and Botanical Gardens. Amputation occurred due to infection, frostbite, and trauma. Many of these people did not survive.

The signs of amputation have been found in prehistoric bones from the Neolithic era. Saws of both stone and bone have been found, imitations of animal jaws with teeth. Höllander (1915) has been able to do an amputation in six minutes with these saws. During the Bronze and Iron Ages, metal saws and surgical instruments were used.

In the Talmud, several references are made to amputation and artificial limbs. A cosmetic fiber arm prosthesis about 2,000 years old has been found buried with an Egyptian mummy with a deformed hand. Elective amputations were done for gangrene or for the removal of mutilated limbs (Friedmann, 1972).

The Greeks and Romans were acquainted with surgical, congenital, and traumatic amputation (Fig. 3).

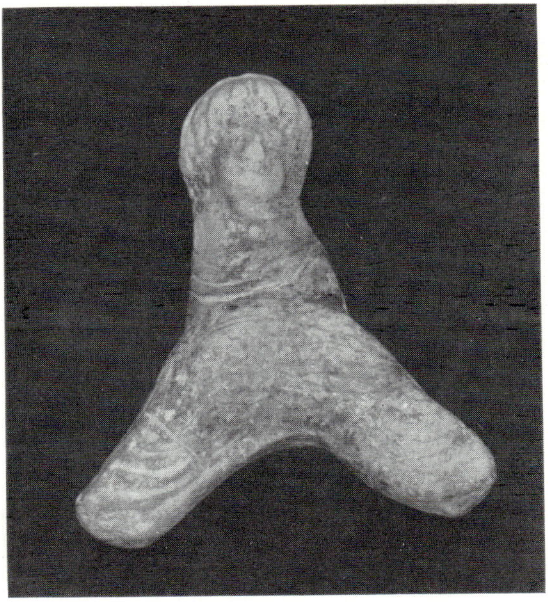

Figure 3. Graeco-Roman mold-cast figurine, Gerasa, Jordan, showing congenital bilateral abrachia. From the author's private collection.

Punishment for crime often consisted of amputation of a limb. In the Arabic countries, for example, punishment for theft consisted of amputation of the right hand. Among the Bedouin, eating is done with the right hand from a common bowl, while the left hand is used for toileting. Amputation of the right hand for theft meant excommunication, since the thief could not eat with other people. It is still done.

Amputations were performed during pre-Columbian times by Indians of the Americas. The best record that is available is from the pre-Incaic time in Peru from 1500 B.C.E. onward. Amputation was done as punishment by the Moche. We are sure of this because of their representative, realistic pottery (Fig. 4) (Friedmann, 1972).

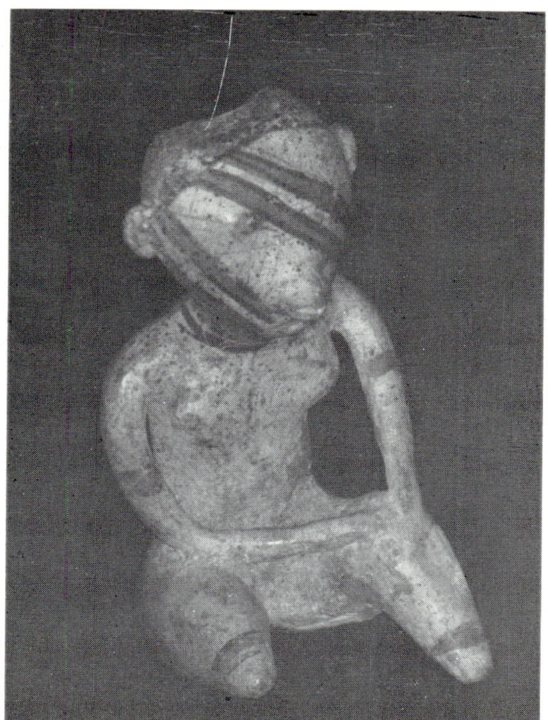

Figure 4. Chinesco-style, post-Classic figurine, Astatlan, northwest Mexico, 800 to 1200 C.E., showing congenital terminal hemimelia, knee-disarticulation type. From the author's private collection.

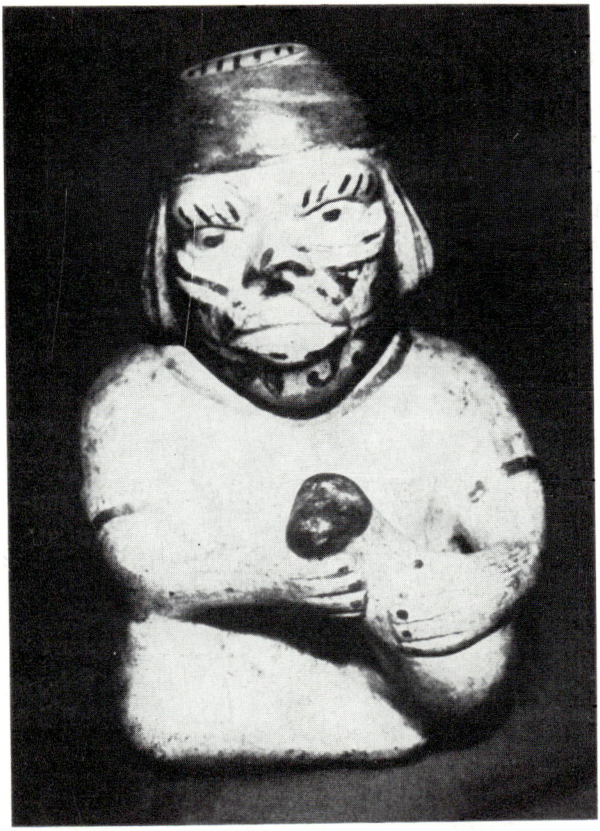

Figure 5. Mochica II, Peru, north coast, showing stump end with granulation tissue, 200 B.C.E. to 0 C.E. From a private collection, Lima, Peru.

Three laws were enough to rule the theocratic pre-Incaic empires: Do not lie; Do not steal; and Do not be lazy. Transgression of these rules led to more severe punishment in the upper classes, on the presumption that they were more responsible for the upkeep of the moral standards of the community.

Lying was punished by excision of the patient's lips and nose. Amputation of a foot was done as a punishment, most likely for laziness. The punishment for theft was amputation of the hand. If, however, a man could prove that he stole because he was hungry, he was let free, and the village chieftain was punished in his place. The theory was that it was the job of the village chieftain to assure that no one in his care went hungry.

The amputation was done in guillotine fashion. Bleeding was rarely fatal. The patients are demonstrated functioning after the amputation. It is not known whether a tourniquet, ligatures, or cautery were used. Some wounds were closed, but others were allowed to granulate (Fig. 5). There are claims that ants' jaws were used to hold incision lines together. This technique is successful, but proof that it was done in ancient times is not available.

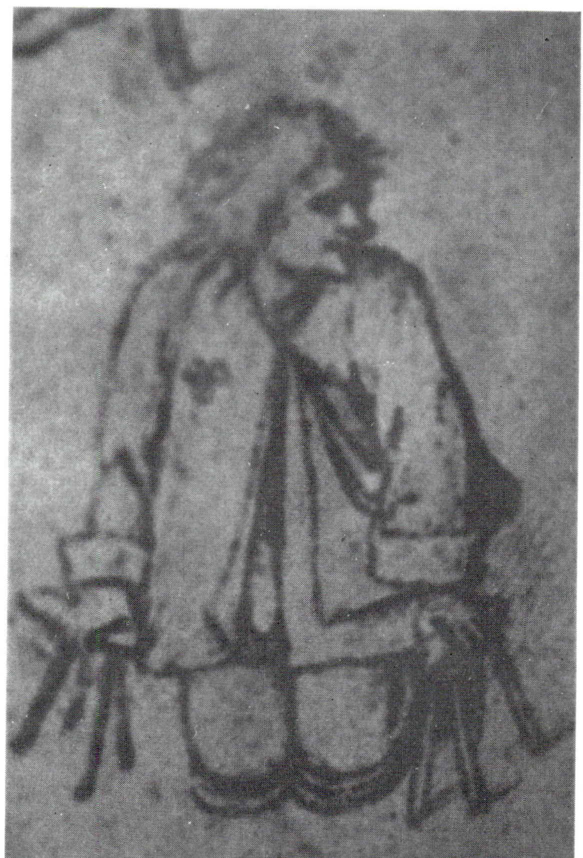

Figure 6. Drawing by Jerome Bosch, the Netherlands, showing a man using leather or wood knee protectors for below-knee amputation with two short crutches. Circa 1500 C.E.

The surgeons of primitive eras used anesthesia from various plants, such as nepentag, opium, Indian hemp, mandrake, henbane, and hemlock, etc. Antiseptics such as smoke, honey, wine, niter, and, later, hot oil, were used.

Paré reintroduced the ligature which had not been used since the time of Celsius. He did the first recorded disarticulation of the elbow joint (1536).

Wilhelm Febry of Hilden, Cologne, 1593, first recommended amputation above the diseased part of a limb. Johann Ulrich Bilguer (1720-1796) recommended in 1761 that conservative surgery of the joints and amputation through the joints be performed, rather than higher amputation. This was before the time of Fergusson, Syme, and Brodie. In 1781, Doctor John Warren of Boston did the first American shoulder disarticulation. James Syme (1799-1870) did the first successful amputation at the ankle joint in 1842.

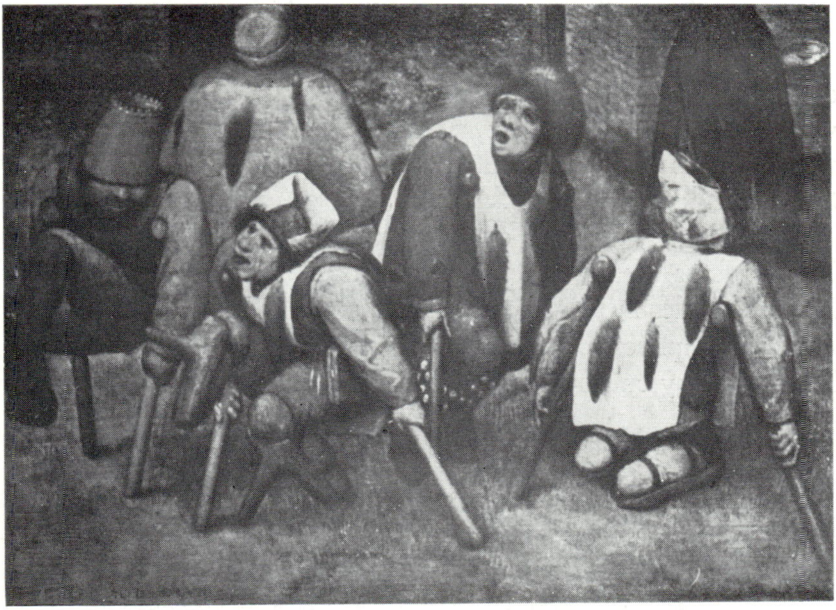

Figure 7. Painting by Pieter Brueghel, the Elder, *The Cripples,* demonstrating bilateral below-knee amputees using various knee protectors and early forms of below-knee prostheses and early crutches. Courtesy of the Louvre, Paris.

Prostheses were developed much earlier for the lower limb amputee than for the upper for obvious reasons. Survival requires the use of a leg to walk on, gather food, hunt, and escape from danger, even in the unilateral amputee. The unilateral upper-limb amputee could survive without a prosthesis.

The lower limb prosthesis has been known for well over 3000 years. Originally for the bilateral amputee, it consisted of leather or wood protectors for the knees (Fig. 6). The crutch was invented, consisting of a simple stick to assist with walking. At first, this did not have an axillary piece or handle. It soon became apparent that holding on to the straight stick was inconvenient. An axillary bar was added (Fig. 7). To free the hands, a resting device, probably an open trough, was attached to the stick, to release one hand for function while standing (Fig. 8). Later, this trough was closed, making the first socket with a crutch tip. The upper part of the crutch was then eliminated. The lower part of the crutch became the pylon. Suspension was by means of straps or by holding with one hand.

The earliest Peruvian prosthesis used was self-constructed and consisted of a wooden cylinder, possibly with soft cloth inside with a band around the top, presumably to hold it on. The cloth would soften the shock of walking on the sharp edges of the tibia and fibula (Fig. 9).

Aristophanes, the fifth century B.C.E. Greek author, has a part for an actor wearing a prosthesis in his comedy, *The Birds.* Herodotus described an artificial limb made by Hegesistratus who was imprisoned and confined in stocks when, in 484 B.C.E., he escaped by cutting off his foot in the stocks. When the wound

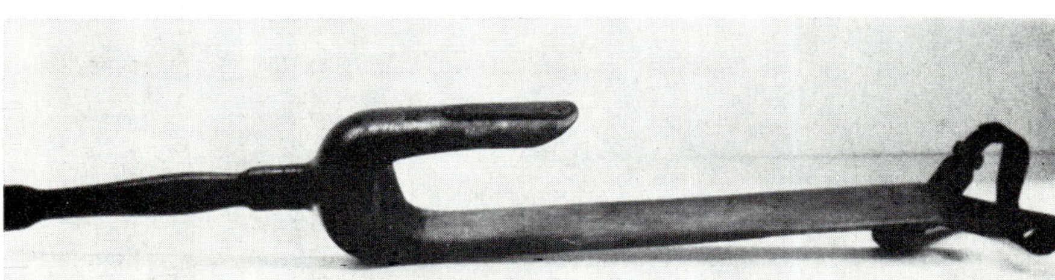

Figure 8. Early open peg-leg prosthesis with open area for kneeling. Courtesy of the Wellcome Museum, London.

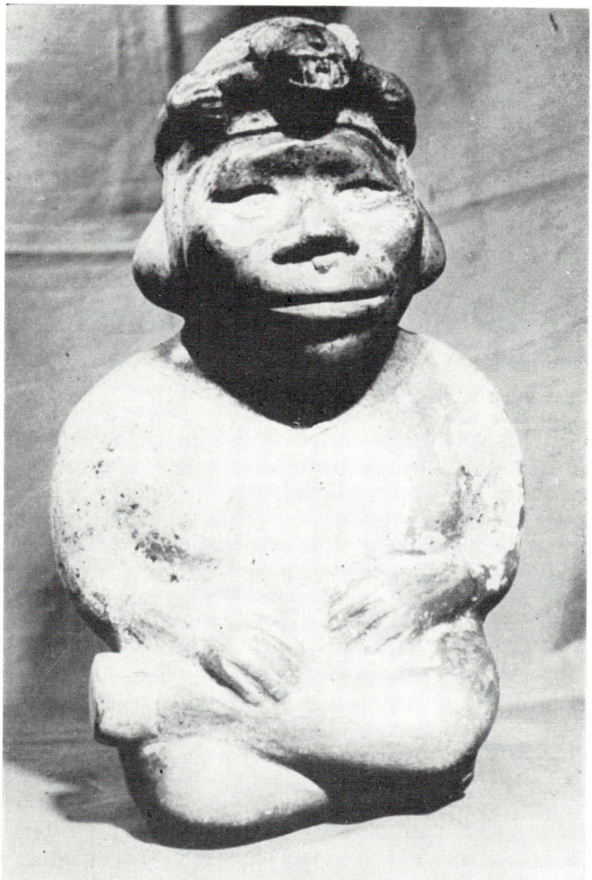

Figure 9. Mochica III, north coast, 0 to 200 C.E. Figure is ankle-disarticulation patient with wooden ankle protector on stump, usually lined with rags. From a private collection, Lima, Peru.

healed, Hegesistratus made himself a wooden foot that he used for ambulation.

In the Royal College of Surgeons in London, there is a prosthesis found in Italy, which has been dated to the Samnite Wars of 300 B.C.E. During the Second Punic War 218 to 201 B.C.E., an artificial hand was worn in battle by the Roman general Marcus Sergius.

Among primitive African societies, if a man was unfortunate

enough to lose a leg, he generally walked with a tall stick or fashioned a crude peg leg from the branch of a tree. The peg leg is extremely functional. The first recorded advance came during the Middle Ages, when armorers built iron artificial legs to be used in battle by the knights. This was especially important, since evidence of infirmity was evidence of loss of a previous battle, a disgrace. These were cosmetic lower limb prostheses. When the knight came home, he used either the crutch or an above-knee peg leg.

The best illustrations of below-knee devices are by Pieter Brueghel the Elder (1529-1569 C.E.). In *Christ Driving the Money Changers from the Temple,* a bilateral below-knee amputee is crawling with protective pads on his shins. In *The Fight Between Carnival and Lent* he shows one amputee with a contractured below-knee stump walking with axillary crutches; one below-knee amputee with a peg leg; and a bilateral ankle disarticulation with severe hip and knee contractures. In *The Netherlandish Proverbs* (1559), he illustrates a Syme amputee wearing a kneeling prosthesis. In *The Cripples* (1558), two have ankle disarticulations and artificial "limbs," wooden shin protectors held on by straps. One wears, in addition, an anterior post that brings the angle of his shin to about 45 degrees (*see* Fig. 7).

Jerome Bosch (1450-1516) did sketches of amputees using crutches and prostheses (*see* Fig. 6).

By 1564, the famous Doctor Ambroise Paré described an above-knee prosthesis with a fixed equinus position, adjustable socket, a controlled knee lock, and other engineering principles still used. This development did not arise *de novo,* but had a number of antecedents. He described a kneeling knee peg leg and an artificial hand with the fingers given full range of flexion and extension and controlled by cogs and catches with springs.

The most famous upper-limb prosthesis was the iron hand worn by Count Goetz von Berlichingen, who had lost part of his right arm at the siege of Landshut, Bavaria, in 1504. The hand had separately articulated fingers that allowed him to close his hand over his lance and remained locked until they were manually released. General François de la Moue also wore a metal hand activated by the normal extremity. Such hands were lockable holding devices. Some were operated by cables activated by the fingers. Mechanically they were ingenious, but functionally they were poor (Fig. 10).

The earliest use of a functional upper extremity prosthesis activated by distal body motors through a harness seems to have been designed in Germany in the early 1800s.

Verduin, a Dutch surgeon, in 1696 devised a below-knee prosthesis with a wood foot, a leather-lined copper socket, and a thigh corset with the external knee joints.

The leg made for the Marquis of Anglesey, England, was constructed so that the knee extension plantar flexed the foot, while flexion dorsiflexed the ankle. It was modified and brought to the United States in 1839 by William Selpho. The principle is now used in a hydraulic leg. Beaufort made the padded kneeling prosthesis with a rocker foot. The principle of the rocker foot is incorporated into the keel of the Solid Ankle Cushion Heel (SACH) foot, as well as being used for "stubbies" for bilateral Above Knee amputees.

The Bly leg (1858) contained a functional ankle allowing

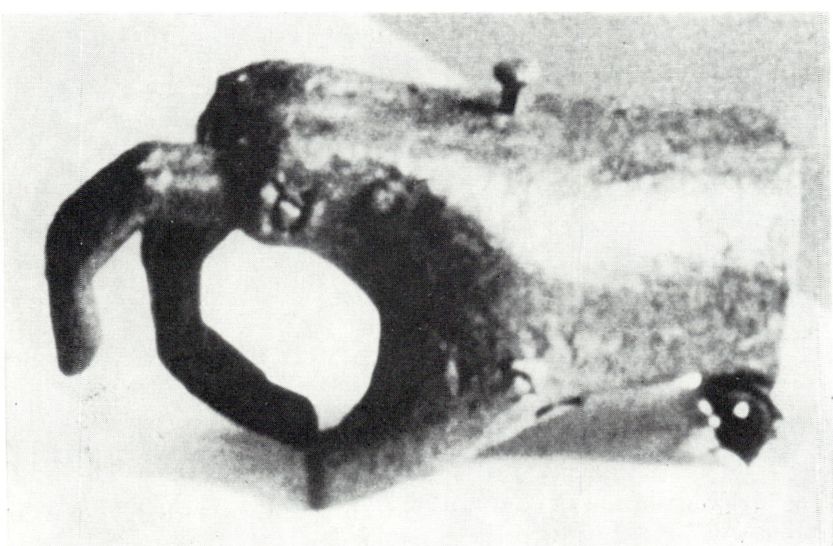

Figure 10. Medieval iron functional hand of unknown date and provenance, Yugoslavia.

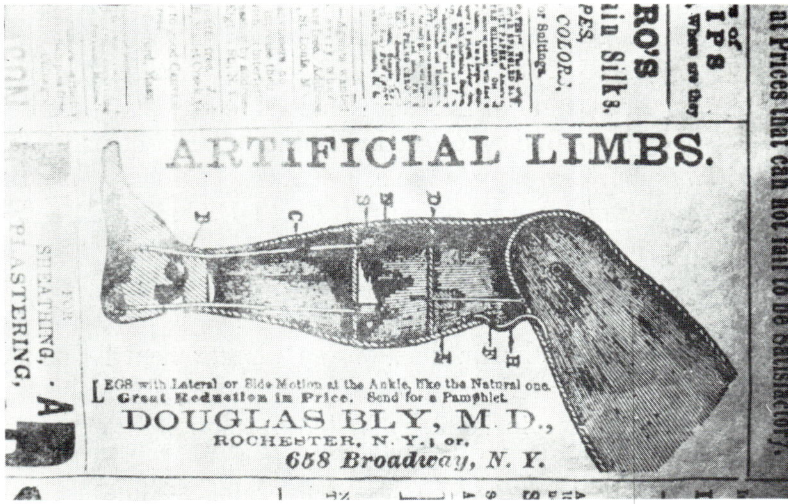


Figure 11. Newspaper advertisement for Bly leg, invented 1858, with lateral motion, as well as dorsi- and plantar flexion.

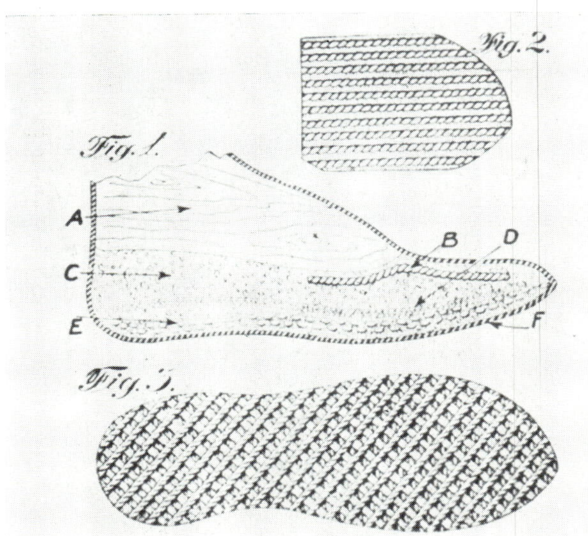


Figure 12. Marks rubber foot, invented 1863, revised 1921, the forerunner of the SACH foot. Courtesy of A. A. Marks Co., New York.

lateral motion, as well as plantar and dorsiflexion (Fig. 11). The Marks rubber foot (1863) revised in 1921 is very similar to the modern SACH foot in function and design (Fig. 12). In 1863 C.E. Parmalee patented a suction socket for the above-knee amputee, a polycentric knee joint and a foot that had three sets of articulations for five toes, along with an ankle that permitted some rotation.

The first known study of the psychic phenomena in those who

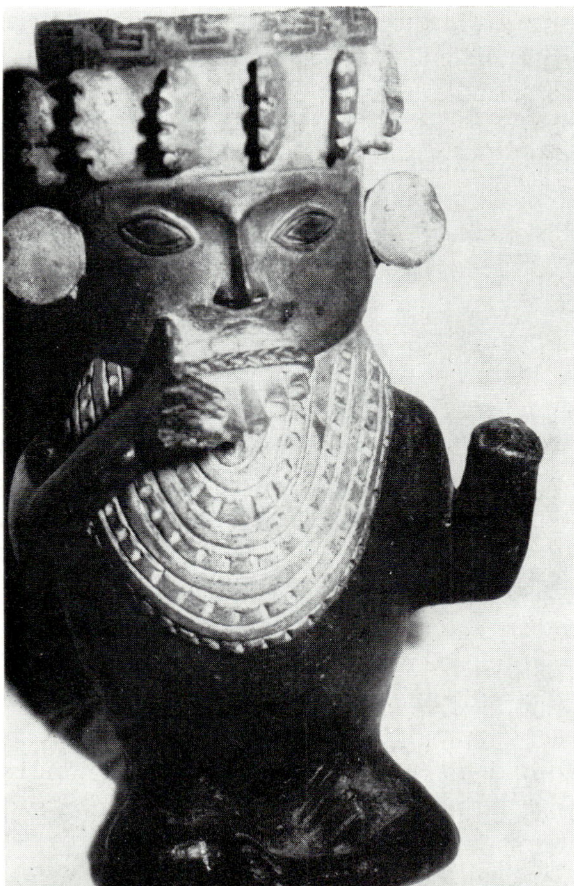

Figure 13. Chancay figurine, Peru, central coast, 900 to 1470 C.E. Figure of punitive amputee of the hand playing the pipes of Pan with one hand, probably begging. Courtesy of the Guggenheim Museum, New York.

had undergone amputation was done by Silas Weir Mitchell (1829-1914), who described phantom limbs and the changes that meteorological conditions cause (1877). He also discussed the psychology of the amputated person in *Injuries to Nerves and their Consequences* (1872).

The involvement of society with the amputee was intimate from earliest times. Society prescribed amputation to worship a god or as punishment. The rehabilitation of the amputee was generally ignored or left to him. Some amputees tried to hide the deformity. Until the sixteenth century, an artificial limb was made by the patient himself. After that, special mechanics, often former armorers, made limbs full time or as a sideline. These were made without prosthetic prescription, according to the ideas of the mechanic. It was rare for there to be mutual thinking about the rehabilitation of the amputee until Doctor Ambroise Paré, who worked with an individual called *The Little Lorraine,* to design artificial limbs.

The vocation of most amputees was begging. Many of these amputees were treated as criminal outcasts, and rehabilitation was not considered (Fig. 13). It is only since the later part of the nineteenth century that true teamwork attempting to get the patient back into society was used. This depends upon an attitude that each individual's happiness is of worth. The team approach can offer the amputee a maximum of productivity and happiness.

Social pressures are such that the majority of the world's amputees still receive care that is at best haphazard. It rarely involves a group of dedicated individuals working together for the benefit of the amputee. It is regrettable that the majority of surgeons doing amputations worldwide have little concept of team rehabilitation. They have only a minor interest in and appreciation for the newest advances in amputation surgery, prosthetic techniques, or social reintegration.

This is the challenge to all of us. How amputees are treated in the future reflects on our civilization and on our concept of rehabilitation: Our actions today will be tomorrow's history.

## Chapter II

# GENERAL ASPECTS OF AMPUTEE PSYCHOLOGY

### Introduction

PSYCHOLOGY is often neglected or glossed over in most works dealing with the rehabilitation of the amputee. This is unfortunate because, in my opinion, emphasis on this subject is necessary. Treating the psychological problems faced by the amputee often has more significance to his life than the quality of the surgery or the nature of his prosthetic device. Training in the broad sense implies, most of all, dealing with the patient's emotional state. Because most of us feel at a loss with these problems, we tend to relegate them to the "back burner" and deal with them by ignoring them. Unfortunately, the amputee cannot ignore them. The disability entailed by amputation either of an upper or lower limb is far more the result of individual and social attitudes than it is with loss of function. While functional problems are generally discussed in terms of loss of physical ability to do certain activities, almost all amputees agree that they have far more difficulty dealing with people than with things. It is the loss of ability to relate psychologically, socially, sexually, and vocationally that inhibits amputees most.

### General Psychic Responses to Amputation

Responses to an amputation depend on many things. Self-pity, anxiety, shock, grief, anger, and frustration are universal. They are not amenable to significant modification. While loss of a limb is always a misfortune and handicap, since it can occur in many circumstances and for many reasons, each can provide a different emotional context. For some people it is a relative blessing, if the limb has been nonfunctional, painful, or ugly for a prolonged period of time, or if its loss kept them from further combat, with its risk of death.

Many patients report disbelief that they were to become amputees or that their limbs had been amputated. Almost all report shock. Prior talk about the expectation of shock is helpful in diminishing it. The shock is most severe when seeing the stump for the first time, especially since they feel the phantom sensation. Fear for the future and panic with compensatory rage and anger are frequent later. Suicidal impulses, grief, self-pity, and despair are almost invariable. If the patients had pain prior to the amputation, they may have a transient sense of relief and happiness. Many avoid reporting their revulsion at looking at the stump. Feeling deformed is common. Disgust at the thought of one's own body being mutilated is difficult to relate. Simpson (1959) says that none of her patients reported feelings of shame or guilt. This might be an artifact of the specific questions posed. Some patients look on loss of the limb as punishment. It is assumed that this is a result of feeling real or imagined guilt (Thorp, 1972).

A number of amputees commit suicide either in an obvious or a covert manner. Resnik (1970) reports that a ten-year-old boy who underwent quadruple amputation for Waterhouse-Friderichsen syndrome attempted suicide. After the amputations, the patient received very little medical attention. Psychological support was slight, from a student nurse. The patient manifested the usual depression and hostility, refusing to eat or take medication. He stated that he wished to die. After psychiatric consultation and follow-up, the fear of abandonment that preexisted the amputations diminished. The neglect was reportedly based on the physicians' guilt concerning their indecisiveness and confusion.

An amputee has the same few alternatives open to him when confronted with an obstacle to his functional performance, as do we all:

1. Retreating, i.e. avoidance of the task
2. Circumvention of the difficulty by compensation, through use of remaining extremities and abilities, either with or without a prosthesis
3. Surmounting the obstacle, if this is possible.

The last is the least feasible of the techniques. An amputee ordinarily uses his/her prosthesis and remaining extremities to best advantage to circumvent any difficulty arising in the performance of the tasks he wishes to do.

The reactions of men and of women to amputation are approximately the same, but sex roles modify the ways the reactions are expressed. There are a number of factors to be considered when discussing the psychological adjustments to amputation and prosthesis. These methods of adjustment to a problem are not different in the amputee than in the normal individual. The patient's desires and drives must be satisfied, and the means for satisfaction are essentially the same as in the normal individual. The patient's basic personality determines the severity and duration of each of the reactions to both amputation and to prosthetic use. Depression is probably the most frequent reaction to limb removal. This can be considered as normal, unless it is extreme and long lasting. It should be combatted by an active all-day program and chemotherapy. If the patient becomes resigned to the amputation, s/he may eventually make efforts to improve his/her function with the use of a prosthesis. When there is a feeling on the part of the amputee that someone else may have contributed to his/her amputation, extreme resentment may result, which may affect adjustment not only to the amputation and prosthesis, but to his/her entire life as well. The anger is often non-specific and should be ignored. The patient may withdraw into himself. Depression and withdrawal are more commonly associated with the elderly and with unstable, insecure individuals, frequently of diminished intellect. More commonly, but not universally, people with higher intellect tend to substitute one form of gratification of desires for another. This occurs especially with the young.

*Obliteration* is the denial of any form of handicap. This may take extreme forms and is usually limited to patients with a mild to moderate disability. These people may become proficient in various types of activity in order to prove that they are not handicapped. This should be encouraged, as a special skill or talent improves a persons self-image and compensates for the loss of self-esteem incurred by the limb loss. *Overcompensation* or *substitution* is an extreme form and can occur even in the markedly handicapped. This individual resents segregation or feelings of being different. The depressed person welcomes segregation and becomes self-conscious, sensitive, and suspicious. Most amputees resent sympathy, but have a deep need for empathy.

Patients with guilt feelings tend to be more interested in cosmesis than in function. Excessive cosmetic concern may, in addition, be a function of the society in which they live and their ethnic background. In most societies, the disabled form a distinct minority group with all of the problems of other minority groups. They frequently form beneficial clubs to help and commiserate with each other. Feelings of inferiority are almost universal. The patients are frequently looked upon as lepers by normal individuals, who often do not wish to associate with an amputee or other handicapped person. Those who do associate with amputees too frequently are overly solicitous and helpful and frequently damage the amputee's adjustment by refusing to reject excessive demands of the amputee in a normal way. Some aggressive individuals may make excessive demands upon other people, some of whom are afraid not to accede to the demands of the amputee.

The adjustment to a prosthesis depends upon the patient's personal adjustment to amputation; upon the basic personality of the amputee and his/her integration of the prosthesis into his/her personality structure. A prosthesis may be considered as assisting in personality reintegration in a number of ways.

The artificial limb helps to restore the body image. Normal individuals view themselves with four normal limbs whose extent is circumscribed, more or less, by the skin. This is ordinarily modified to include clothing and commonly used objects. For instance, when driving, each person includes the size of the automobile into his "body" image. This allows him to maneuver the automobile in space without damaging nearby objects or the automobile. Body image has limits that are not exactly the actual limits of the body. There are educational, psychological, and neurological changes in body image. An artificial limb returns the patient's body image toward normal by replacing the missing part. The exact process by which this is accomplished emotionally is not known. Some amputees are able to totally integrate their prostheses into their body image, feeling "naked" without their prostheses. A frequent reaction to amputation is a revival of the castration fears of childhood, with a feeling of "not being a whole person."

The prosthesis is considered by most amputees a means of concealing the amputation. This is most common in those ashamed of the amputation because of guilt. When a patient feels that an amputation is punishment for sin, either real or imagined, then he attempts to disguise this sin or the fact of amputation with a prosthesis, which must be as cosmetic as possible. This also holds true in the case of children with limb-reduction deformity. Concealing a disability is advantageous. It helps the amputee to a more normal appearance, avoids reactions of pity, and aids in identification with a normal populace.

When the amputee views the amputation as castration (a lack of ability to perform), the loss of a precious part of oneself, this tends to be somewhat ameliorated with the use of a prosthesis. Stress on use training is the best treatment. This is related to the loss of any body part and even to death of a friend or family member. Those amputees who reject the amputation as unacceptable to their self-concept make poor use of any prosthesis. As research continues and externally powered prostheses utilizing proportional electromyographic controls become more efficient and natural, we hope that acceptance by arm amputees of the prosthesis into the body self-image becomes easier and more crucial to successful use.

Amputees describe themselves differently after amputation than before. This is not only in a physical sense, but also emotionally. They describe themselves as being less active, energetic, and adventurous and more awkward. These are realistic estimates of changes in their state due to fear, less normal function, and their use of energy for limb activation.

There is a very real belief in all societies that suffering and illness are visitations from heaven as punishment or as a means of atonement for sin. This primitive feeling is shared by the amputee. Barker et al. (1953) state that various scholars have proposed the following to account for the psychological effects of physical disabilities: (1) compensation for inferiorities; (2) narcissism arising from uniqueness and discomfort; (3) lack of normal expressive action, such as play; (4) concentration of emotional energy onto the amputated limb; (5) anxieties transferred to the amputation; (6) parental blame in congenital anomalies or early amputation; (7) guilt to compensate for hostility toward parents; (8) a body image that differs significantly from reality; (9) efforts to achieve social acceptance in the face of social rejection of the disabled; (10) demanding dependent behavior when in an overly protective situation; (11) variability of behavior in response to inconsistent outside attitudes; (12) goals above the possible level of achievement because of outside economic, social, physical, and parental pressures; (13) the conflict between compensatory activities and withdrawal; (14) the attempt to accept disability as punishment for sin; (15) aggressive behavior to compensate for "unjust" treatment by nature or persons around the patient; (16) problems of self-image; (17) the amount of acceptance of the disability; (18) reconciling personal and social value systems; (19) problems with cultural acceptance of amputation; and (20) intergroup dynamics.

Some of the intervening variables leading to or affecting adaptation of the patient to amputation, either congenital or surgical, have been the following, according to Wright (1960):

1. Value system of the patient
2. Effect of the amputation on status
3. The patient's need for social and personal acceptance as a worthwhile individual
4. The patient's self-image
5. The behavior of the individual and the relationship of those standards of behavior which the patient approves of, and his own actions
6. The acceptance of a change in value systems, which leads to acceptance of the reality of limb-loss
7. Revision of the patient's expectations and goals when

s/he realizes that there is a discrepancy between what had formerly been expected and what is now possible

8. The use of grief as a means of catharsis that allows the patient to begin the process of adjustment to amputation
9. The identification by the amputee of positive goals and self-characteristics allowing the assumption of identification in a positive way with persons and ideals, which can be accomplished after amputation
10. Motivation toward reinstatement into society.
11. The ability to cope with loss, rather than succumbing to disability

Chapter III

# PATIENT REACTIONS TO AMPUTATION

## Adult—Acute Postoperative

When amputation is due to trauma, the patient has the amputation almost before s/he knows it. The traumatic amputee has many emotional reactions somewhat similar to other amputees, but to a different degree. Immediately after a traumatic amputation, patients are in shock, pain, and frequently under sedation, and are really not too aware of what is occurring. Surgical consent in this situation is meaningless if it is from such a patient.

If the amputation is delayed for any reason, patients feel a variety of emotions, including depression; suicidal urges, even in those who have never considered suicide before; anger both at themselves and others; fear; worry; and in certain cases, guilt. Some amputees are glad that the accident did not kill them or was not worse than what it was, but this feeling soon disappears in most of them. Fear of death and of the future is universal. Whether a patient feels guilty or not depends upon whether the accident was due to his negligence. In terms of the feeling of guilt when the accident was not of his doing, the situation is much more complex. For those who believe in God, the reaction may be one of the expressed or unexpressed feeling that God has punished them for some sins, by inflicting upon them an amputation. On the other hand, many very religious individuals resign themselves to the fact that the amputation is "God's will" and manage to eliminate the guilt. Those who do not believe in God may feel that the amputation is punishment for sin, but do not articulate the feeling well. There is almost a primitive, magical quality to this feeling. They feel the limb loss is part of their general societal maladaption. Primitive peoples view all illness as evidence of social maladaptation.

After a few days, the patient begins to fear for his future and this is manifested by anxiety, self-pity, and depression. Intermixed with this is hostility against himself, the medical team, and the cause of the amputation, whether this is military, an accident, or illness. The hostility should not be responded to in kind. The hostility is frequently masked by oversolicitousness and overfriendliness to the medical team. This seductive behavior is an attempt to "buy off" unpleasant treatment. If he is lucky enough to be in a hospital with a large amputee population, he then slowly begins to become involved with the problems of rehabilitation and becomes knowledgeable about care of the stump, the use of prostheses, and the problems of a return to life in society. There are many fears centering around interpersonal relations: familial, vocational, social, and sexual. The fears require frequent discussion and work to remove the realistic problems the patient faces. After some period of time, the patient may become extroverted, especially if young. These patients occasionally manifest their anxiety by joking about the amputation and trying their manhood with aggressive, boisterous behavior (Brown, 1970). There is often anger at the staff, which may be a reaction to the patient's fear of the unknown.

Even patients who desire amputation because of severe pain and disability and who actually beg the doctor to take off their limb have an initial tremendous shock and sense of loss once the amputation is done. Most patients who lose their limb due to disease feel a sense of relief to get rid of the problem that was plaguing them, despite their regret at the loss. Their ambivalence confuses them.

Many amputees feel that it is of great importance for a similar amputee to speak to the patient both before and after the amputation. This is useful to alleviate fear and promote emotional catharsis. It is only later when s/he has time to reflect upon the consequences of amputation that the patient becomes afraid and depressed because s/he has lost an important part of himself. A period of mourning is universal after the loss of a limb. This is frequently followed by minimizing the importance of the amputation and by joking about it. It is only after the latter phase that more serious considerations about the future begin to creep into the mind and actions of the amputee. It is then that social, vocational, and educational planning should be stressed.

The amputee who has been normal up until the time of the

accident is suddenly faced with the fact of major disability and does not have the time for prior emotional preparation. His immediate reaction is one of shock and a complete loss of personality integration. The fact that the amputation is sudden and unexpected and that the psychological reaction to disability has not been formulated offers a unique opportunity to the physician and other members of the amputee team to intervene and to help the patient make an adjustment in the most appropriate manner. This is much more difficult to do in the elderly.

## REACTIONS TO AMPUTATION—CHRONIC

### Adult—Preoperative

The reactions to amputation vary, depending upon differences in the person's antecedent emotional state. If the amputee has an amputation of a lower extremity because of vascular disease, this has usually been preceded by a long period of illness and disability, frequently with pain. The patient has had time to ponder the fact that the circulation in his lower extremities is progressively decreasing. The patient has begun to accustom himself to the fact that he is disabled by the pain and is partly used to viewing himself as a disabled and limited person.

#### *Chronic Occlusive Arterial Disease*

Ordinarily, when gangrene is present, the patient subconsciously appreciates that ablation is a possibility. It is advisable to bring this possibility to the patient's consciousness even before overtly mentioning it to the patient. This is best done by pointing out to the patient the severity of the problems that he is having, such as severe pain, ulceration, or gangrene. In the presence of pain, it should be pointed out to the patient that prolonged symptomatic relief with narcotics cannot be continued, since addiction to narcotics is serious. Since painful phantom is more common with prolonged pain, amputation should not be delayed too long. Immediate amputation, however, should not be considered unless uncontrollable infection makes it necessary. A delay of a week or two allows psychic and physical adjustment to occur.

It is quite important to discuss with the patient the importance to his general well-being of an appropriately timed amputation. A detailed discussion of the benefits, such as the relief of pain and the improvement in function with prompt fitting of an artificial limb, is important. If an early or immediate prosthetic fitting can be offered to the patient, it may reassure him. Prolonged delay in trying to save the foot may decrease his ultimate physical and emotional function, perhaps permanently. In the end, the patient almost certainly comes to a major amputation, due to the natural course of the disease. This may convince him to delay no further.

A frank discussion is frequently avoided by both the surgeon and the patient, and this is detrimental to both. A realistic brief discussion of the advantages and disadvantages of each course of action should be an important part of the decision to amputate.

In contrast to Warren and Record (1967), I feel that the possibility of amputation should be mentioned, in most cases, where there is the slightest possibility of its occurrence. I maintain that the avoidance of mentioning this as a possibility until "all doctors concerned with the case feel that it is indicated" does the patient a disservice. A frank discussion of the strenuous efforts to save the limb leads to an appreciation by the patient of the possibility of amputation, if the efforts fail. It gives the patient time to adjust mentally. In my experience, patients try to avoid the realization that amputation is a possibility, and if presented with that recommendation suddenly, a short time before the amputation is contemplated, it may prove to be overly traumatic.

It is important that the patient understand that no amputation is done until everyone is agreed that there is no reasonable recourse but amputation. Comfortable, safe walking is the aim of all concerned. The patient should realize that the retention of a painful or useless extremity is detrimental to his personality and physical well-being. A prompt amputation with a good prosthetic fitting usually allows the patient to participate in many of the activities he enjoys that are denied to him as long as he retains the painful, functionless limb.

It has been my experience that the possibility of amputation tends to bring to the foreground those aspects of personality one would expect that an adult patient has outgrown. Usually, these are patterns of emotional response reinforced by stress during early childhood. Prior to surgery, most patients tend to suppress aggressive and hostile actions toward all staff members and especially toward the surgeon. This appears to almost be a plea for a decision not to amputate, since amputation is viewed as punishment. The surgeon is viewed as the instrument carrying out punishment. Being solicitous of the surgeon's well-being seems to be an attempt to "buy off" the "punishment." The surgeon should not be seduced into waiting too long.

Prior to elective surgery, patients need reassurance of their level of functioning after surgery. Because the patient wishes to minimize the severity of functional loss, when the surgeon comments that the patient will be "almost normal after amputation," the patient and, sometimes, the family obliterates the word "almost." Prior to elective amputation, there is frequently the denial that the condition is really serious enough to require amputation. I have had a number of patients delay permission for amputation long past the time when it became manifest that it was inevitable. In these cases, there is no choice but to wait. It is important to discuss the dangers with the patient and with the patient's family.

The desire to retain ties of affection with family and friends, as well as with the medical team, and the value placed upon the medical staff's respect and affection play no small part in convincing the patient to undergo surgery. A conscious use of this phenomenon helps the surgeon get the patient to do what is necessary for his well-being. Patients requiring amputation, like all patients undergoing the threat of a serious procedure, vacillate before giving consent, unless they are emotionally prepared for the procedure or given an adequate opportunity to adjust themselves to it. The situation must be presented to the patient as a definite decision about which there can be no question. One of the best ways to do that is to make an attempt to save the limb, thereby demonstrating to the patient that everything that can be has been done to save the limb without amputation and that the decision to amputate has been taken reluctantly. When the unequivocal recommendation to amputate is given, the patient is in a better psychological framework to accede to the amputation.

When a patient is extremely fearful, there is little benefit in prolonged discussions of training procedures and detailed discussions of the pros and cons for any decision. The more anxious and fearful the patient is, the less is heard of what the medical staff is saying. The slightest chance remark sets the patient off into his fantasy world of misinterpretation. It is for this reason that clear-cut decisions must be presented to the patient in the simplest and most objective manner possible. The patient should be presented with the necessity for amputation by the surgeon and physiatrist together. Any facts presented during this session other than the necessity for amputation will probably not be remembered by the patient, due to the psychological shock of hearing that his limb has to be amputated. In spite of this fact, it is very important that the physiatrist immediately point out that to replace the lost limb, a new limb is to be provided, if the patient seems to be a candidate for an artificial limb.

As the time of amputation nears, the patients become more dependent upon authority and exhibit little overt aggressiveness. After the amputation, as rehabilitation increases, more and more aggressiveness is exhibited. It is a medical truism that as the patient's physical status improves, so his complaints increase.

Holling (1972) states that when the surgeon and patient have agreed that amputation is necessary, the operation should be carried out as speedily as possible, because for most patients, the period of waiting is one of extreme emotional stress. He states that he has seen two cases of perforation of a peptic ulcer in patients awaiting amputation. He suggests that tranquilizers should be used, in addition to analgesics before and after amputation. Holling claims that some patients refuse amputation despite the need and most careful preparation. Coercion should not be attempted, because the patient who is determined not to have an amputation can live with the bad limb in an incredible fashion and can often manage to get from the bed to the toilet without assistance, while after amputation, he frequently needs assistance. In addition, Holling points out that amputation is associated with significant morbidity and mortality from pulmonary embolism, myocardial infarction, and other causes sufficient to deter one from pressing amputation onto a reluctant patient. Legal as well as medical adverse reactions may ensue.

In cases where the decision has been delayed and the time before amputation is prolonged, the reaction is somewhat different. There may be disappointment and grief at the loss of the limb after a prolonged attempt to save it. There may, in a few cases, be relief at the final solution to a prolonged problem.

It is extremely important for the surgeon to have periodically stressed that he is making every effort to save the limb, but that the possibility of amputation is present in case of treatment failure, once amputation seems to be a potential outcome. In this way, the patient has time to get accustomed to the possibility of eventual amputation. When the time comes for amputation, the patient still expresses grief and disappointment. His reactions are relatively minor, compared to the patient who is presented with a final decision and who has not previously thought of the possibility of amputation or, at least, has not formulated it fully in his mind.

When the possibility of amputation is brought up to a patient in whom it seems very likely, it should always be coupled with a statement that, though an amputation may be needed, the patient's life will be changed, but not markedly. With the use of an artificial limb, he will be able to be happy and useful.

A frequent error is to tell the patient only that amputation may eventually be needed. If it is left this way, without stress on postamputation rehabilitation, then amputation becomes the "bogey man" for the patient, and becomes the mark of failure of reconstructive and therapeutic attempts. In this eventuality, the patient considers an amputation the failure of the surgeon concerned. Unfortunately, the surgeon also sometimes considers that amputation is the final evidence of his failure to save the limb. Thus, both the patient and the surgeon are despondent over the presumed failure and tend to ignore the positive results of an adequate treatment program. Both the surgeon and the patient must be made aware that the failure of certain reconstructive efforts and the resort to amputation is not failure, but only a level of success slightly below that of reconstructive procedures with adequate rehabilitation.

In patients with malignancy, delay is not advisable. Most patients should be told that they have a malignant tumor, and that the limb needs to be removed to attempt to save his life. A few patients do not want to know and permit amputation without questioning why it is needed, because they are more afraid of the term *cancer* that they are of amputation. The diagnosis should not be pressed upon them—they know it anyhow. People refuse to see the obvious as a defense, and we should not breach that defense, as we can substitute nothing better for it. Only when treatment is rejected is it necessary to force the diagnosis on the patient. Sensitive clinical wisdom is needed to distinguish who should be told from who should not and to find the proper words for that individual.

Physicians, surgeons, therapists, and patients must be brought to the awareness that, in the care of patients, death is the only ultimate medical failure, and even that is sometimes a blessing. Very close to this failure is the lack of restoration of maximal potential function to an individual. When the patient and surgeon consider that amputation is the mark point of failure, functional failure is frequently assured. If the patient considers amputation as a lesser degree of success, but still successful in that it can restore him to a relatively functional, satisfying life, then the patient and the surgeon and other members of the amputee clinic team have been successful.

When an open amputation is necessary for drainage of an infected wound, it is important to explain early the necessity for a second amputation to provide a good stump. If this is not done, the patient and his family frequently assume that the secondary procedure was due to the failure of the surgeon to do a "good job" during the first amputation. This may give rise to litigation.

The patient frequently has many questions that should be answered. The questions should be encouraged in as natural a way as possible by the person who has the best relationship with the patient and, in the particular case involved, seems to be best in dealing with these problems. The patient frequently wishes to know whether his life will be shortened by the amputation. This can usually be answered by indicating that his life expectancy will not be shortened by the amputation itself. His life expectancy depends upon other factors, such as the cause of the amputation and other diseases, etc.

The patient frequently worries about the effect of amputation on his employer and fellow employees, how this relates to his job, and how his family and friends will relate to him as an amputee with a changed ability to function in many ways. Bringing out this universal fear by leading the patient to ask a question is the best method for explaining to the patient that his acceptance by the community, family, and employer depends far more on his adaptation to the amputation and the prosthesis and his ability to function, than it does on the amputation itself. It is sometimes helpful to stress that many famous successful people had disabilities—Franklin Delano Roosevelt, poliomyelitis; Helen Keller, deafness and blindness; and Galileo, epilepsy. It should be affirmed to the patient that his ability to succeed and his value as an individual depend not upon his limbs as much as upon his willingness to work, dependability, intellect, and personality. I use the phrase "Any animal has better legs than you or I, but our unique humanity comes from what we have in our heads and hearts." Stress is thus placed upon those qualities which remain after, rather than upon those faculties diminished by the amputation. In this way, the amputee is encouraged to look ahead, rather than backward.

The question of sexual potency is not frequently raised but is often a fear. Sexual potency is only diminished when the psychic concomitants of amputation cause a depression that involves sexual function. Rarely diabetic neuropathy or vascular occlusion can be causative. Some amputees later become "sexual athletes." It is not unknown for divorces to occur, because the marital partner is unable to accept any type of disability. In these cases, the marriages were usually unstable before the disability, and the amputee must be brought to the realization that he is usually as well off without this partner. On occasion, patients inquire whether congenital amputation is hereditary. One can only answer that in some cases it is, but in the majority of cases, it is not. Genetic study should be done in all cases to alleviate the fear and to be certain. I have had a number of patients ask whether acquired amputation becomes hereditary. Frequently, there are now questions by parents of congenital amputees whether some medication given during pregnancy could have caused the amputation. Unless there is definite evidence, the answer should be no. However, it is important that pregnant women be given as few medications as possible during pregnancy, especially during the first four months.

Patients frequently want to know how much disability they will have. This, of course, depends upon their state before the amputation. The best way of answering this is to have an amputee with a similar situation talk to the patient. Patients are remarkably ignorant as to what an artificial limb can do. Some expect it to have all of the attributes of a normal limb, including sensation. General guidelines should be given to the patient by someone knowledgeable as to what he can and cannot expect to be able to do after the amputation and fitting with a prosthesis and with training.

A detailed discussion of the various types of prostheses early is inadvisable. The reason for this is that the patient is so emotionally involved in his reactions to the need for amputation and his concerns with his future that any detailed discussion of specifics is ignored by the amputee. General terminology and predictions and, if possible, showing the patient a similar patient with an artificial limb who is functioning at a moderate level of success are encouraging. The use of a "professional amputee" or one who is an extremely good user is inadvisable, since it may lead to excessive expectations. The personality of the patient and the demonstrator should be taken into account before introducing the two. Having patients wait in a common area for an amputee clinic is best, so an appointment system should not be used. Grouping physical therapy and occupational therapy sessions so that amputees are treated together and can see each other's struggles and successes is best. Patients are remarkably uninformed and must be given complete instructions, e.g. the care of the prosthesis, when it is and is not to be worn, what purposes it may and cannot serve, the inadequacies of present prostheses, and the difficulties that the individual will have in adjusting to the prosthesis.

Presentation of a prosthesis alone I have found to be more detrimental than helpful, in contrast to the experience of some.

Detailed descriptions of the surgical procedure or of rare surgical risks are psychologically harmful to the patient and should be avoided. This is somewhat difficult to reconcile with current medical-legal tendencies in which there appears to be a trend toward informing the patient of all of the possible consequences of any course of treatment about to be undertaken. The physician and surgeon thus can be criticized equally for under- as well as for overinforming a patient.

Patients who exhibit a great deal of anxiety and fear prior to amputation, with extreme agitation, difficulty in sleep, restlessness, who are not responsive to usual doses of sedation, and those who cancel surgery or leave the hospital against medical advice have the high level of anxiety persist after amputation. These patients are often preoccupied with events that frighten them, both before and after surgery. The most frequent compensatory mechanism is oversolicitousness towards the staff and expression of their gratitude and admiration in the most profound terms. They attach themselves firmly emotionally to the staff and make great demands. They are usually friendly and cooperative, but have intermittent periods of hypochondriasis. They need much reassurance. Prior to surgery, they try to distract and resign themselves to the inevitable. Those individuals try to consider the secondary gains to be obtained from the amputation, both economic and emotional. Their needs for support are great. Reassurance of these people is extremely difficult. In this group, preoperative information about surgery and postoperative care does not seem to modify the amount of anxiety, in contrast to patients with a low or moderate level of anxiety.

In some cases, excessive anxiety may be due to misleading information from others, but more often is due to preexisting psychoneurosis, which most often cannot be alleviated in the available amount of time. Panic can usually be alleviated somewhat by tranquilizers. Psychotherapy is of little use at this stage, in my experience. For these patients, a minimum amount of information about the surgery is probably best.

Burgess et al. (1971) speak of the importance of the immediate postsurgical prosthesis in improving the psychologic state of the amputee. In doing so, they point up clearly the importance of the psychological attitude of the surgeon toward amputation. Whether or not the immediate postsurgical prosthesis is used, the attitude of the surgeon and the amputee rehabilitation team should always be hopeful, while being realistic. There is rarely need for unlimited pessimism with these individuals. Burgess and his colleagues state that the attitude of many surgeons toward amputation really is,

> Intangible but definite psychological benefits should result from immediate postsurgical fitting with ambulation. Prior to surgery, in elective amputations, the patient can be told that he will be "up the next day or so and on his feet." A hopeful rather than a negative approach to surgery is thus accomplished. Most elective surgery connotes a state of improved physical well-being. The totally destructive nature of an amputation confronts the patient with irreparable psychological disaster, in many instances. This is particularly noted among older people who, looking at their remaining years, are concerned acutely about helplessness and dependency. The rapid transition from limb loss to function bespeaks hope. This motivation can make the difference between effective rehabilitation and failure.

It is important that elective amputation also connote a state of improved physical well-being. The gangrenous limb that saps the strength, both physical and psychological, of the patient and inhibits his normal life is being removed, to be replaced with a functional, nonpainful, and nondangerous prosthesis. The patient will be "up the next day and on his feet," even without an immediate postsurgical prosthesis, since the patient should be up as early as possible walking in the bars or on crutches. Amputation is not "totally destructive," but a stage in reconstruction, whether or not the immediate postsurgical prosthesis is used. Indicating to a patient that he will not be helpless and dependent if he participates in a rehabilitation program is what is most important. The use of the immediate postoperative prosthesis is one method of convincing the patient that the amputee rehabilitation team means what it is saying, but is by no means the only method by which this feeling can be conveyed to the patient. Motivation is important and often makes the difference between effective rehabilitation and failure. It is the attitude conveyed that is important and not the specific means by which this attitude is conveyed.

### Adult—Postoperative

After the initial reactions, a slow or rapid coming to terms with the amputation occurs. Even after seeming initial acceptance of the situation, occasionally patients revert to inability to accept it. They may go into frank psychosis, alcoholism, or the use of drugs. One patient was reported by Simpson (1959) to have said that he still has the feeling that some day he will be well again (without the amputation), twelve years after amputation. I have had similar cases.

Amputees, like the rest of us, resist facing the realities of their situation some of the time. The amputee must become reconciled not only to the fact that the extremity is gone, but that he is less complete and attractive physically; he will suffer discomfort, inconvenience, and expense; there will be limitations to locomotion or hand function; and much more energy expenditure is required and his choice of recreation curtailed. There may be a need to start a new job, social discrimination, embarrassment in dealing with other people, and possible recurrent medical problems. It is a universal trait to minimize one's handicaps. It is unpleasant, but we must deal with reality as it exists, and not with the world as we would like it.

One common way of protecting against the emotions aroused

by amputation is to deny the significance of the amputation by overcompensation. This may be done by excessively hard work or excelling in recreational activities, etc. Peter Strudwick (1972), with bilateral foot absence, is a marathon runner. It is as though by an act of will one could force fate to reverse itself. The limbless feel that it is helpful to think of the amputation in relative terms. By comparing their own misfortune to that of others, they feel that their situation might have been worse. Being together with other amputees apparently greatly facilitates thinking about one's own injury in relative terms. Pursuing positive goals helps handle negative feelings. A religious attitude or faith in either a Supreme Being or in medicine may be helpful. Some people compare the loss of a limb to other more common physical infirmities, such as aging, the use of hearing aids or eyeglasses, or false teeth. It helps to put it in perspective, and this kind of discussion makes it a more familiar and more tolerable situation.

The patient may have neurotic problems because of protracted pain or fear of death due to malignancy prior to amputation. In addition, he frequently has had prior operative procedures and been withdrawn from his previous environment of work and family life. He is fearful of what will happen to him, economically, socially, and sexually. In addition, the patient has psychological problems due to sensory deprivation, since a highly sensate organ is removed. The sensory input from the skin of the foot and proprioceptive input from the multiple joints, muscles, and tendons of the foot and ankle and the receptors from the muscles of the calf are removed.

The patient has a psychologic need to replace his real limb. This is manifested not only in the acquired amputee, but also in the congenital limb-reduction deformity. There is a great seeking for an actual replacement of the lost limb even in mature, intelligent adults. This results in a desire for a transplanted limb, cosmetic limbs for lower extremity patients who cannot walk, and in one case of the author, a mature, intelligent congenital amputee who requested a false limb that would look as normal as his remaining leg, not when he walked or was seated but undressed, when he went to bed with his wife. This "neurotic" but normal behavior in the face of absence or abnormality of the body part may cause various types of disturbances, frequently sexual. The more the prosthesis deviates from the functions of the absent limb, the greater the psychic abnormalities. My wife had one congenital amputee whose mother asked my wife whether transplantation of limbs was successful. The reason she wanted to know was because she and her husband were seriously considering having another child for the sole purpose of removing the new born child's arm, transplanting it to the remaining limb of the living child and killing the child they were planning to conceive. While this proposal is fortunately rare, it illustrates the absurd lengths to which people are prepared to go to achieve their idea of normality either for themselves or for members of their family.

Some patients are very critical of prostheses that do not closely mimic the appearance, feel, and function of the normal limb. Even temporary devices are criticized, because they do not have a cosmetic cover. These amputees tend to be highly vulnerable to the attitudes and emotions of others. Doctors are authority figures and become heroes or villains. The first visit of a wife, children, or other family members may cause patients to lose control of their emotions. The prosthetist may bear the brunt of the patient's emotional reactions. Expressions of sympathy and offers of help may arouse emotional crises, since they contribute to self-pity and a feeling of being crippled. There seems to be some ambivalence about receiving assistance.

After the initial and subacute reactions, chronic aftereffects psychologically are anxiety, loss of trust in others, inhibitions, hostility, and fears. There is very real irritation and disappointment about minor things that the patient cannot do or that emotionally hurt.

After surgery, a single, detailed explanation of the rehabilitation plan is almost worthless to the patient. Shortly after surgery, a simple explanation in a conference with the patient and family present should provide a general outline of the plan of rehabilitation. The outlines of the plan are spelled out at that session, but individual steps of the plan are delineated periodically at follow-up visits and related to the general plan as the patient progresses. Each person can only really comprehend one or two new concepts every few days. The purpose of the general outline is to present an overall picture. It will have to be repeated a number of times during the patient's rehabilitation for optimal effect. Each time a new element is added, it should be related to the total context of the plan delivered at the family conference. The proposed next step, following the one about to be started, is usually presented, so that the patient begins to understand the relationship of each step to the total program. The aims of the total program are frequently brought before the patient and are primarily determined by the patient's own life goals.

Postoperative emotional reactions depend on the individual. Some persons are isolated and fearful, especially the more elderly or less educated; they withdraw and become isolated almost to the point of becoming hermits. This isolation is much more severe than the functional loss would require.

Younger and better educated amputees and those with mild to moderate functional loss may overcompensate by becoming "professional amputees." These people deny that any disability exists. They engage in sports and many other activities of the non-amputee and, in fact, may spend considerable time proving how well they can function as amputees. These people demand treatment from others as a nonamputee. This is an excellent reaction, provided it is not taken to extremes. Arm or leg amputees can participate in many sports with major or minor modifications. There are ski races for amputees and many athletic activities, including competitive athletics. Unilateral amputees of either upper or lower extremities can play basketball, baseball, golf, bowl, run, dance, and ride horseback, etc. Bilateral upper- and lower limb amputees can learn to swim with ease.

The amputation is sometimes used as a weapon to control others. The person uses his disability for secondary gain, economic as well as social. The amputee can use it as a weapon with which to control family and friends. If this is carried to extremes, the amputee may lose both.

Still another reaction to limb loss is the compensatory form:

The more severely disabled, intelligent amputee realizes that while his goals may remain the same, he must take different means to attain his goals. A person's goals of leading a useful, relatively independent life, in which he can earn a living and earn the respect and affection of others need not be changed. The means of attaining these goals and the specific jobs available to him may need revision and restructuring. These are generally not too difficult to accomplish, if the patient is willing to adapt to the required changes. Help from the vocational counselor, social worker, and psychologist is most fruitful here.

It has been noted that patients who undergo an amputation and expect to be totally disabled after amputation tend to become euphoric, when they appreciate that total disability is not in store for them. But, patients who expect to be normal after amputation and to be able to resume their previous activities unchanged tend to be depressed after amputation. The time of fitting a patient with a prosthesis and the psychological approach to the patient thus become crucial.

If a patient is told that he will be able to resume his normal life or if he interprets the remarks of the staff in that light, his tendency toward depression is greater than usual. However, if he expects to be totally dependent, his reactions after amputation tend to be euphoric. The value of early prosthetic fitting can thus be appreciated. The time delay between amputation and the beginning of functional return is much reduced. This allows a more rapid appreciation by the patient of both the difficulties and the opportunities that he has before him. It allows the patient who thought he would be totally disabled to see that he can walk. To the patient who thought he would be normal, it allows reality to be tested rapidly. It is important that the patient's concepts of his function not be distorted by inadvertent comments of the medical team. While ideal gait is desired, if the person is satisfied, only minor corrective efforts should be undertaken.

As the date of amputation recedes in time, there is a period of self-pity, during which there is an increase in self-indulgence. This self-indulgence frequently reflects the patient's prior methods of coping with stress. A patient who used food to relieve emotional stress in the past tends to overeat. Dietary control is almost impossible to maintain. This may have serious consequences in terms of socket-fit maintenance. Those who indulge in cigarettes, alcohol, or drugs may revert to these habits. Neurotic symptoms are expressed more during this intermediate stage than before or after. This usually occurs from the second through the fifth week after an immediate postoperative fitting, during the third through the sixth week of an early postoperative fitting, or in the first through the fourth month or even later during delayed fitting.

If the patient is overly encouraged concerning the potential of rehabilitation prior to or immediately after surgery, his emotional reactions to the disappointment are frequently expressed not only in grief, but combined with rage, expressed not only to the medical staff and family but inwardly as well, with self-punitive behavior, hopelessness, and lowered self-esteem. Along with grief and rage, if the patient's functional state is less than what he inwardly expected, the blame is frequently placed upon the medical personnel, especially if the patient perceives any deficiencies in the care he receives. Thus, if one must err in estimating a patient's future potential, it is better to err on the side of conservatism and not overoptimism. One of the prime foci of rage in this type of person is the feeling of being abandoned by the medical staff. This feeling is especially acute when the physician does not see the patient for a period of time and does not designate a surrogate whom the patient expects, knows, and respects. Visits from the family are extremely important on weekends and when the physician cannot visit the patient.

Individuals demonstrating very little fear or anxiety prior to elective amputation tend to display more anger and resentment after, especially if they have much pain or difficulty in adjusting to the use of the prosthesis. A moderate amount of anxiety and fear prior to amputation seems to minimize postoperative emotional reactions. Most amputees harbor a great deal of suppressed hostility. It is kept hidden in fear of retaliation and is usually expressed only in the company of other amputees, trusted friends, or while intoxicated. This is why most survey type studies do not show it.

The above reactions pose some interesting problems for the surgeon and the rest of the amputation team. The so-called good patient who shows no fear prior to surgery is precisely the patient who is likely to be complaining later about his treatment being poor, careless, and unprofessional. This person should be provided with enough information to arouse a slight degree of apprehension. It is useful, in this group of patients, and to a lesser extent in patients with moderate fear, to alert them to some of the minor inconveniences, unfamiliar sensations, and the slight amount of pain experienced after surgery. While they should not be frightened, a somewhat realistic picture should be presented. A general outline of the work involved in the rehabilitation program is advisable. This should be presented over a period of time and not all at once. Vivid descriptions are frightening and should be avoided. Ventilation of fears is desirable. This is not usually possible for the medical team during ward rounds. It is best for the surgeon or one of his surrogates to do this. It is seldom that this patient needs psychological or psychiatric assistance, although a psychiatrist with experience with amputees can be invaluable.

Among the psychological problems of the amputee, it must be remembered that the peripheral vascular disease patient has impairment in both lower limbs and in his cardiac and cerebral circulation as well. It is possible that the patient's main complaints after surgery relate not to his amputation stump and prosthesis, but to the pain and fear of losing the opposite limb occasioned by disease in that organ or of the real possibility of heart disease or stroke. In the cancer patient, fear of death is usual.

Patients undergoing amputation for malignancy are often grateful for the amputation, as they view it as lifesaving. They rarely refuse amputation, except as part of a general refusal to accept the diagnosis. To these patients, provision of a prosthesis early is vital to give them hope of cure. Delay makes them despondent.

It is advisable to encourage the patient to discuss his fears and anxieties; he must feel that freedom of communication is possible. This process is best done in short periods over a number of days, rather than in one or two long sessions. The doctor must be perceived as being not in a rush.

The psychological implications of amputation are great, since the amputee internalizes society's attitudes. They include loss of self-esteem, loss of completeness of the body image, loss of respect for one's appearance and functional ability, and inability to relate to oneself, one's spouse, and one's family, friends, and employer in a normal manner. An amputee must learn to adjust his self-concept, so that the deformity and the prosthesis are incorporated into his body image. The amputee, in meeting a new person, benefits from having a prosthesis that is not too noticeable, since it allows the patient to begin the relationship so that the new person can relate to him as a person, rather than looking through him and being solely aware of the artificial member.

Psychologically, the term used in amputation for the remaining member, *stump*, is objectionable. It evokes in the mind of the amputee and of others a tree or branch that has been cut off, leaving a ragged, deformed, unsightly remnant. It is far better, when talking with the amputee and his family, to refer to the "remaining part of the arm" or "residual leg." When asking to see the stump it is better to ask the patient to "let me see your left leg." Since the term *stump* is so common, the patient undoubtedly hears the term used frequently. After a time, he should be introduced to the term, preferably in a nonthreatening manner and time. Unfortunately, there is really not an adequate substitute term at this time, so that a significant effort to use another term would not be fruitful. It is hoped that someone will propose such a term in the near future.

In my opinion, deep psychic intervention is rarely needed, provided there is a well-trained staff willing and able to give proper guidance to the patient. There are patients who need active psychiatric care by someone experienced in the care of amputees and the reactions to amputation. These patients are usually older, withdrawn individuals, frequently from the lower socioeconomic and educational strata. They usually become more depressed, irritable, and aggressive. They sometimes drown in a sea of self-pity. Fortunately, this is not common.

Knapp (1968) believes that the services of a psychological counselor should be used. In my experience, it is the rare psychologist or psychiatrist who has the experience to deal with these problems effectively. The additional threat of having to deal with the psychologist or a psychiatrist may add to the threat of amputation and may be overwhelming for the patient, especially the elderly; for many of them, the referral to a psychiatrist is tantamount to considering them psychotic. If, however, the physiatrist and/or surgeon do not have the time or inclination to perform this necessary duty, then the services of a competent psychiatrist or psychologist are vital. The reason that I feel that the physiatrist and/or surgeon should do this is that they have a better knowledge of functional end result and can bring more reality into the patient's situation than the psychiatrist, unless an exceptional one is available who has had experience in dealing with amputees and prostheses. Psychiatric help is of greatest benefit after the initial shock of limb removal and prosthetic fitting has worn off.

### Training—Adult

Predictions of the functional consequences of varying amounts of physical loss are often inaccurate, since they are overshadowed by psychological factors, especially the patient's perception of his disability. Most patients estimate their abilities and disabilities poorly. Since these perceptions are inaccurate, the patient's responses are inappropriate when viewed in terms of reality. Thus, the treatment of the amputee assumes two foci: (1) diminution of physical loss by appropriate medical care and (2) revision of unrealistic ideas and attitudes.

Some of the human needs that cannot be completely satisfied after amputation are physical function, visual and auditory cosmesis, comfort, minimization of energy cost, achievement, economic security, respect, and status (Fishman, 1959).

The doctor's attitude is extremely important. The patient must feel that the doctor is exerting himself to do his very best for his patient, at any age and with any medical condition, including cancer. No patient is too old for a prosthesis without a trial, unless there are definite medical contraindications. The patient becomes very depressed after an amputation, although there may be an initial period of euphoria. This depression is deepened, if the doctor is not hopeful or does not allow the patient to see whether s/he can use a prosthesis. Fitting of a prosthesis is the next most emotionally laden experience associated with the amputation. Reality must be faced, and some of the illusions about an artificial limb making them "as good as new" have to be confronted. The pain, frustration, and energy expenditure of learning to use a limb are particularly disturbing to those individuals trying to forget the loss of a limb or minimize its importance They may want to abandon the effort temporarily. At this time, complaints about poor function, excessive weight, and poor cosmesis are frequent. Consistent use and success diminish some complaints, but rare individuals are not satisfiable, looking for a *status quo ante.*

Amputation involves a loss of body image as well as a body part. Care must therefore be psychological, as well as physical. A purely engineering solution is inadequate. The patient and the prosthesis ideally should form a single unit in which the interface and interaction between the individual and the prosthesis are of prime importance. During and after prosthetic training, psychologic help is most valuable, no matter by whom it is given.

Because the lower limbs are not as immediately in the field of vision as is the face or the hands, amputation of a leg is somewhat less obvious and, therefore, less psychologically damaging than loss of an upper limb. It is the *obviousness* of a loss that is most detrimental. If, however, there is a cosmetic defect because of poor gait noise, malodor, or a hard texture in the prosthesis, then cosmesis is diminished, and attention is called to the fact that the patient is an amputee; social and psychological problems magnify. *Static cosmesis* relates to visual, olfactory, or tactile noticeability at rest. *Dynamic cosmesis* refers to the appearance in motion, that is, trick motions in grasp, excessive "body English," gait deviations, and auditory noticeability.

All amputees have a fear of the unknown, and each member of the amputee clinic staff must take the time to explain the problems involved in terms that the patient can understand. Explanation is only effective for those capable of understanding. Patients ask questions of therapists, nurses, and aides more frequently than they do of the physician, since they feel closer to and see them more often. It is important for the therapy staff to convey these questions to the physician for explanation where there is any doubt of the adequacy of the answer. The more active the therapy program both before and after the surgery, the less time there is for the patient to dwell upon his fears and to become despondent. It is for this reason that an active therapy program should be started at the earliest possible time, and certainly, no later than the day after amputation. This will usually involve the unimpaired extremities only, at the beginning, but it involves the patient in doing something with a view toward his future function and partially eliminates the universal feelings of worthlessness and a feeling that life has been ended by the amputation. The amputee in a hospital that does not have a significant amputee load with whom the new amputee can relate and maintain contact or one discharged from a hospital without an amputee clinic with frequent follow-up manifests further anxiety under pressure, as the realities of adjustment to the amputation and to the world outside the protective walls of the hospital close in on him. He has no one to whom he can turn for answers. If an active rehabilitation program is not provided, this anxiety and depression may last a lifetime, resulting in an emotional cripple. This is far more disabling than the limb loss.

The importance of the amputee team in helping the patient work through the problems posed by the disabilities in combination with his personality, motivation, and the support given by his family and society in general, are crucial in smoothing the transition to the nonamputee environment. Try to ensure that the patient learns to consider the amputation as of far lesser importance than other aspects of his life, including not only general health, but integration with society. Other amputees are very helpful in giving a new amputee guidance, if they are chosen wisely.

In dealing with civilian amputees, we are dealing with the normal distribution of society skewed towards the older age-group. Each clinic has different experiences, depending upon its accidental or voluntary preselection of patients. In each group there are some patients so highly motivated that they succeed with or without training. Aid to these patients is accepted with gratitude and rapidly incorporated into the patient's life. Any aid given is utilized to the maximum, and frequently, the patients develop new and improved methods of rehabilitating themselves. Some of these patients become "professional amputees." They can do remarkable things with their prostheses.

At the other extreme of the spectrum are those patients who were functionally marginal or inadequate prior to their limb loss, and the amputation has definitely not improved them. The patient cannot cope with life after amputation. For these patients, there is no way of modifying the situation. Minor attempts to produce a productive individual should be tried, but failure is usual. It is very easy to prejudge certain individuals as belonging to this class and not give them a chance. I feel this is unjust, since some individuals who appear to fall into this category, if handled properly, can become useful individuals. This requires considerable judgment and skill. Some patients take a longer time to demonstrate their potentials. I believe in giving each person a trial where it is feasible. After a relatively short time, if there appears to be no possibility of success, I do not continue to push. I believe in reviewing failed patients at least every six months, in order to determine whether progress can be made with further work. A delay in formulating tentative end goals increases the cost to the patient and to society, both economically and emotionally. The goals must be expressed and discussed with the patient, and often revised as the patient is known better.

It should be explained to the patient that he must adjust to the limb and vice versa. Changes will be needed for a long time both in the limb and in himself. There will be shrinkage of his stump as he uses the limb. This is expected for at least one year and usually more. He must be told that every time he changes a component in the limb, it will require a period of adjustment, just as when he "breaks in" a new pair of shoes, only more so. It should be explained that he is now bearing weight on parts of the body that were not intended for this purpose, and the skin must be toughened to sustain this weight. He should be forewarned about the muscle aches and pains that he will endure when strengthening his musculature to adapt to new patterns of muscular behavior when using the artificial limb.

One of the most distressing types of patients to work with are those patients who have been told by their surgeons that "you will be almost normal after we fit you with an artificial limb." Most of these patients block out in their understanding the word "almost." These patients frequently become very uncooperative and depressed, as the reality of less-than-perfect prosthetic function impresses itself, as it must, with all present devices.

The reaction to wearing an artificial arm varies with the individual. There are some individuals for whom, culturally and individually, the loss of a limb is psychologically devastating, since it is interpreted either by the patient or by the society in which he lives as punishment by the Divine Being for some sin. In these cases, cosmesis is most important, since it hides the fact of amputation from the public, thereby hiding the sin from public view. For certain individuals, cosmesis is extremely important, not because of their own emotional state, but because of the repugnance that most people have toward an artificial limb or toward disability of any kind. The Latin cultures are extreme examples of cultures that foster this feeling.

Disguising the deformity is done by construction of artificial limbs so that they appear as nearly normal as possible. The use of special devices and tricks such as the use of rings or wristwatches on the artificial limb, the carrying of a briefcase or a handbag on that side, the wearing of gloves and specially tailored clothing, the use of a Band-Aid® on an artificial hand are examples of useful ways to distract attention from an artificial hand.

In cultures in which cosmesis is of less importance, some patients discard cosmetic prostheses after a time, unless they are functional as well. This is because they are heavy, increase perspiration, and are cumbersome. It is for this reason that most high unilateral upper-limb amputees discard any prosthesis. Efforts to increase the utility by externally powering these prostheses are usually futile, because these devices are very costly and inadequately functional to compensate for the excessive weight, cost, and lack of reliability. A one-handed person is almost completely independent in all activities, when properly trained.

In the lower-limb amputee, a similar problem may exist: Frequently, active, young individuals reject the use of an artificial above-knee or hip-disarticulation limb, since they find that the weight and the effort required to learn to use it are annoying. They find that they can use crutches with ease and that this satisfies them. These patients usually later realize that their function and appearance are worsened unless they get an artificial leg. They are often socially less acceptable and less desirable as potential employees, since with crutches, both hands are occupied, and they can carry nothing. With a good lower-limb prosthesis, they can free one or both hands. With these people, prolonged efforts at verbal convincing are futile. One can only hope that, with time, what has been said sinks in. The patient then usually comes and requests an artificial limb. He subsequently, usually, becomes an excellent user. I have had more difficulty with patients demanding artificial limbs who cannot use them than I have had with patients who can use them and who refuse to do so.

An artificial limb is a tool. Like any tool, it must be used properly for the job for which it was designed. Patients who use a limb as a tool frequently incorporate it as a part of their body image and feel "naked" without it. It is the same process by which all of us who drive an automobile "know" the limits of our car and feel as uncomfortable when the automobile's limits are being encroached upon as we do when trying to squeeze our bodies through a narrow space. This incorporation of the limb into the body image tends to decrease the feeling of artificiality when the amputee uses his prosthesis. With poorly suspended, malfitted, or externally powered prostheses, the direct relationship between muscular action and prosthetic action is diminished. The first two should be corrected. We hope the third will not markedly diminish the sense of the prosthesis "belonging" to the body of the amputee. Direct proportional myoelectric control may enhance incorporation. The work on semiburied implant prostheses by Friedmann, Katz, and Siffert (1972) may aid in this process by making the prosthesis a permanent part of the patient physically and psychically.

As the patient begins to learn to use the prosthesis, it is extremely important that he be sent home from the hospital on occasions with the prosthesis, once it is safe to do so. This allows the patient to appreciate those problems that he is having at home and to bring these problems to the staff, so that they can work with the patient to solve them before he goes home for the final time. In addition, this allows the family, friends, and neighbors to see him with the prosthesis and for them to get accustomed to the patient's new circumstances. It allows these individuals to sort out their emotions and reactions, so that there is some stability and acceptance by the time the patient arrives home permanently. In addition, when the patient has progressed in his training program, a review must be undertaken of his job situation, hobbies, and other interests. Amputation affects many aspects of a patient's life, and all of them must be considered.

It is amazing to some of us who see many amputees to realize the extent of ignorance of prosthetic function among upper- and lower-limb amputees. Strangely, even some patients who have worn prostheses for years express the fact that they know little or nothing about how an artificial limb works. There are some amputees who believe they know everything about the functioning of a prosthesis. These people frequently modify prostheses on their own, sometimes destroying them. Prosthetists are the most frequent source of information, followed by other amputees. The family physician is a poor source of information in most instances, since he has little information about the amputee state or detailed information about prostheses. There appears to be a dearth of information given to an amputee by anyone. If instruction is given, it is usually given intermittently, haphazardly, and in a manner the patient finds difficult to understand. This ignorance on the part of patients appears to me to be a significant factor in the mediocre rehabilitative results obtained in most hospitals. Few involve the patient and his family in the process of rehabilitation. Fewer yet make the amputee the central figure in the rehabilitation process.

The reactions of an amputee vary with time. Most patients in a general hospital are not informed of the problems involved in prosthetic usage, nor the availability of care.

It is my experience that the emotional impact of the amputation is so great at the beginning that patients cannot take too much information. The fact of being an amputee must mature in the psyche of the amputee. Most amputees have great expectations from artificial limbs. They often expect them to perform as well or even better than normal limbs, and are not aware of their limitations until after considerable use. They almost invariably conceive of artificial limbs as almost a complete replacement for their missing part. This is especially true in our modern age of technology when patients literally ask, "If we can go to the moon, why can't we have an arm or leg which really functions naturally?" It is good that these expectations occur early in the rehabilitation course. Most patients, if informed too early about the deficiencies of prostheses at the same time that they are depressed about the amputation itself, may have a more severe depressive reaction than is necessary. After the patient's wound is healed and he is becoming accustomed to the fact of being an amputee, then gently and slowly, progressively more facts must be provided to him These facts must include the deficiencies of our prosthetic and rehabilitation armamentarium. The best way of showing a patient the difficulties of using an artificial limb and the deficiencies in the limbs themselves is experience with the limbs. This is best done by provisional temporary prostheses.

Most leg amputees benefit from seeing similar patients further along in their therapy early. This should not be done too soon for amputees of the hands. Seeing another amputee walk with an artificial leg is nowhere near as frightening as having your hand amputated and seeing a patient using hooks the next day. Most patients with hand amputations live a fantasy life that either replaces their original hands or gives them a substitute equivalent to a hand. The patients get emotionally stronger while their wounds are healing. This gives them some time to begin to face reality. The realities must be presented to the patient slowly and, preferably, by example, since if the realities are presented too rapidly, they may become overwhelming and cause the patient to break down emotionally. If the process is slow enough, then when a patient is presented with hooks, the well-adjusted patient will say to himself, "Well, I have to make it with these. These are now a part of me and I have no other choice."

Most patients, both male and female, need someone in the therapeutic team as a strong father-friend image, whom they can look up to and respect. This depends not only on the individual's knowledge of the details of the care needed, but on his emotional and intellectual strength. The strength must be modified by a felt impression of being a real friend to the amputee.

Amputees lose status in society. The loss in status may be due to economic factors, but, more importantly, is due to the lack of regard of society for the disabled. This attitude is usually reflected in the amputee's attitude towards himself. As with other minority groups, amputees overtly look upon themselves as the same as other individuals. Their inner feelings belie this general statement. When questioned carefully by someone they like and trust, amputees share society's negative view of them. This is a significant and all-embracing fact of their existence. Because society's values are internalized, the Negro and the amputee both appreciate that race and amputation are pervasive and significant factors in existence. To deny the reality of this factor is comforting to the amputee, but is not a reflection of the reality with which he must deal.

While denied by many amputees, there is no doubt that the feeling of loss is persistent and remains throughout life. In some individuals it is more hidden than in others. This is expressed in self-consciousness and feelings of inferiority, etc. This is made worse by functional decrements or losses, awkwardness, and the visibility of the prosthesis. Education is necessary in order to work through some of the significant interpersonal problems in relating to outside society, including school, job, and dating, etc. Methods of patient education are still in their infancy. We do not know yet the relative efficacy of patient and parent groups, literature, video tapes, and radio broadcasts. There is little doubt, from my experience, that it is beneficial for groups of patients to get together under the guidance of a dynamic and educated group leader. For the child amputee, similar sessions for the parents are beneficial.

Special educational efforts are needed in relation to significant psychological and social events in the patient's life, such as prior to entering school or the first date, etc. These events may require meetings with the school principal, the school teacher, and the parents, and occasionally involving the child. It is important to make arrangements for the child to show his prosthesis to the other children and tell about it and to answer his schoolmates' questions. This does not obviate all problems, since other children will still tease the child about his loss. The problem is much greater for a girl than for a boy, because boys can use the prosthesis to fight with, and this is a way of gaining status among boys. Appearance is of such importance among girls that they really have no compensatory means of gaining status among their peers. While this problem is of importance in all ethnic groups, among certain groups, it is even more important. Among Latins, for example, appearance is of such importance generally that extreme methods are employed to achieve cosmesis, even at the expense of function. Although figures are not available, suicide is relatively high among South American women arm amputees. In many parts of the world deformed-child infanticide is still common.

Amputees maintain feelings of self-worth by denying and

overcoming the physical difficulties and abnormality as much as possible. Amputees deemphasize the disability caused by their physical defects. They place the amputation in the background and do not wish to identify with the disabled. Disabled individuals evaluate their own achievements highly.

Amputees may deny their limitations and claim that they can perform as well or better than nonamputees. This may be a good reaction, especially for patients with minor losses. For patients with major losses, this is usually an adverse psychological adjustment, since the patient, in order to maintain this fiction, must restrict his activity so severely as to constitute a pathological withdrawal from life.

Amputees often deny that the amputation interferes with their ability to get and hold a job, even in cases of very severe functional and cosmetic loss. This appears to be a reflection of their desire for normality and a condition that does not exist. A man with limb absence has difficulty in accepting that he can do less than a nonamputee. This is despite the fact that it takes some extra effort to keep up with nonamputees. This indicates the desire to maintain self-esteem and confidence in the face of severe loss of status and functional potential. Some of my colleagues deny that society has such negative attitudes toward the amputee. The experiences of my patients seem to be typical. Frankness is hard to obtain when one is not similarly afflicted. Denial seems to be a reaction of how the amputee would like to be regarded rather than the way he actually feels. Patients with a poor self-image are generally those with unstable motivation and who are compulsive, timid, hostile, dependent, and rationalize their situations. The patient with a strong self-image generally is more self-assured and confident, and his confidence is deeply seated. Motivation is more steady, hostility is under control, and this patient is outgoing.

The studies of Siller and Silverman (1958) indicate that while 41 percent of their amputees say that they never feel sorry that they are amputees, most of their patients admit to either fantasy or regret feelings when questioned closely. This indicates that, while the amputee tries to deny the effects of amputation, especially the feelings of loss of body integrity and inadequacy, especially to normal people, he cannot really carry it off. Feelings relating to sense of loss are generally related to loss of function. The emotional implications, in my experience, relate little to loss of function, but relate mainly to the obviousness of the loss. The thought of being different from other people is disturbing to most amputees, although it is generally denied when speaking to nonamputees. Only during intimate contact with amputees who have a close attachment to the examiner, such as in a psychoanalytic situation or in the case of someone close and respected, do some amputees admit to their real feelings, such as their fears of sexual and general inadequacy, concern over loss of appearance, and inner fears relating to nonacceptance by normal people. The limbless person often needs to admit these things to himself to compensate for these feelings.

The finest reaction to the amputation is more or less acceptance of the fact and regarding it as a challenge to be overcome. This provides the foundation for prosthetic use success and success in meeting life's goals. If, however, the amputee uses the amputation as a means of justifying his dependency needs or as a means to avoid competition, then the secondary gain derived from these feelings assures that the patient always complains about the prosthesis and blames all of his personal inadequacies and failures on the lack of perfect functioning of the prosthesis. For these patients, the best prosthesis available is not good enough. Many amputees, even with moderately severe losses, reject all prosthetically available items, because they do not approximate the functions of the normal extremity. This occurs especially in unilateral upper-limb amputees and probably reflects their inner decisions to deal with the world as amputees, rather than as nonamputees. I feel that most amputees never totally accept their loss, but learn to deal with it, and this is true, irrespective of the type of treatment that they have received.

Most amputees learn to deny their rejection of the amputee state. They do not accept their loss, and this lack of acceptance is reflected in their distaste and, oftentimes, refusal to associate with other amputees and their discomfort in such association.

Their attempts to deny their amputee status and their feelings of inferiority go very deep, which makes detailed study of this problem extremely difficult. Siller's and Silverman's (1958) figures point this out. Of their patients, 99 percent considered themselves normal people except for a physical defect; 28 percent of their patients considered themselves completely normal, not even conceding the slightest physical defect; only 1 percent of their sample considered themselves as physically abnormal people. In addition, only 38 percent of their sample considered that their amputation made more than a slight difference in their lives, when in fact most of them had a significant modification of their lives, due to this event. Siller and Silverman agree that all of these figures show the extremely strong tendency to reject any hint of abnormality on the part of the amputee.

Amputees are aware that people stare at them and discuss their problems as if the amputee were an inanimate object. Amputees recall how they reacted when they came in contact with disabled individuals before they were themselves disabled. The amputee often considers how he himself thought of the disabled prior to his amputation, in order to reflect on what others think of him now. He thinks of himself as a "cripple," which implies guilt and its punishment, inadequacy in certain tasks and, very possibly, the need to accept charity. These are all reasons for loss in self-esteem.

The younger amputee is usually more adaptable, while the older amputee tends to be rigid in his thinking patterns and less capable of learning. His need for physical function is less, but at the same time, his abilities are decreased. Economic insecurity leads to severe stress emotionally.

It appears that the sense of disability is primarily related to activities. The great dividing line appears to be those patients who can walk and those who cannot. It appears that there is less difference in attitude between a uni- and a bilateral amputee than we previously expected, provided both can walk. The problems are grossly different between walkers and nonwalkers. Those who can walk, irrespective of the severity of their amputation, provided they have normal intellect, appear to do better than those who have great difficulty in walking. The sense of independence is very important for most amputees. Most amputees verbally accept the fact that complete independence is rarely possible for those with walking disabilities. The reason for this is that society places a great premium on personal independence, and walking implies independence. One woman missing both arms and one leg, when asked what limb she would choose if she could get only one back, chose the leg without hesitation, despite good use of her leg prosthesis.

Some amputees display an extreme form of independence. Others exploit their disability and use the amputation to avoid responsibilities. They exploit family, friends, therapists, physicians, employers, fellow employees, other patients, etc. This is a way of avoiding responsibility and frustration. It is a way of controlling other people and also threatening them. Amputees may exploit others, economically, socially, sexually, and educationally. Exploitation may be used as a means of taking revenge on others by limiting their freedom of action, especially through the use of guilt. It may be used as an attention-getting mechanism and an attempt to obtain expressions of love and concern.

What we desire as an adjustment is for the patient to appraise realistically his residual abilities and disabilities and to attempt to compensate for the disabilities in the most appropriate, possible way. Amputees regard a prosthesis as not only functionally desirable in making them more independent and more secure, but often as contributing to their emotional well-being. Even in situations where prosthetic function is not required, an artificial arm apparently is often an asset in giving the amputee increased confidence, which in turn makes him more accepting of the loss and allows him to view the world more realistically. Patients feel wearing of the prosthesis makes them more self-sufficient. Most amputees consider that patients who wear prostheses are less easily embarrassed socially than patients who do not wear prostheses. Unrealistic expectations, later not fulfilled, can interfere with the successful wearing of a prosthesis. This may even be of greater importance than any discomfort.

If patients use a prosthesis, disability is lessened, so they find it easier to accept the fact that they have some disability. They are therefore less shy and more gregarious. They react better to people, either in or outside of the therapeutic situation. Their relationships with their families improve, since they do not feel themselves as dependent and as frustrated. Thus, the decision to reject a patient for prosthetic prescription may be traumatic. If this appears to be the case, consideration should be given to providing the patient with a purely cosmetic prosthesis for psychological reasons. Although such prostheses are expensive, it should be realized that at today's costs, a prosthesis costs the equivalent of less than one week's hospital stay and less than twenty psychiatric interviews. If it appears that serious emotional disturbances requiring treatment will occur, it is far less expensive to provide the patient with a cosmetic prosthesis than to treat the emotional problems engendered by not giving him a prosthesis. If it is dangerous for the patient to use a prosthesis, then a purely cosmetic, nonfunctional one can be given. A distinction must be clearly drawn between prosthesis *wearing* and prosthesis *using*.

Repeated efforts to integrate what the patient is now doing and experiencing with his future is vital. Vocational, along with prosthetic, evaluation and training must proceed. In my experience, a positive attitude as to what the patient can be expected to do is generally preferred, provided it is not overly optimistic.

Experiences with reality are a more positive and believable stimulus to change of opinion than the most expert medical or psychological help. In cases in which the emotional responses of the patient do not seem to be adequately handled without formal psychological intervention, the psychologist and/or psychiatrist may be needed for diagnostic and/or therapeutic purposes. In my experience, the need for this is limited. The psychological and psychiatric staff, however, plays a crucial role in a significant number of ways. The most important are those advisory and consultative situations in which the amputee's milieu needs to be improved. Therapists need to handle the more serious problems of amputees in line with their professional responsibilities. Unfortunately, many psychologists and psychiatrists have very limited experience with amputees and are uncomfortable with them.

Many amputees reject psychological appraisal and help, despite their need for it. If, however, the amputee clinic team is fortunate enough to have a psychologist and/or psychiatrist with special knowledge and interest in the amputee, this may prove invaluable.

The use of a vocational counselor in rehabilitation clinics should be routine: First, a number of amputee patients can be expected to go back to some kind of work. More importantly, the very thought that consideration is being given to having them go back to a functional wage-earning place in society is of great benefit to these patients.

The term *motivation* has been so overused that it is difficult to use in a way that is comprehended by all. It appears to me that each person has special motivations toward comfort, security, and self-esteem. The way in which these needs are met depends upon one's capabilities. It is important that the entire team determine the patient's views of his needs and attempts to relate the rehabilitation process, so that it is obvious to the patient that his needs are on the way to being met in the optimal manner.

Probably the most important predictive determinant that relates to the success of the rehabilitation efforts is the patient's preamputation state, both physical and emotional. Some patients have spent their entire lives looking for a reason to withdraw from a competitive existence. They cease competing after amputation and hide from a threatening world.

Persistence with a patient may result in meeting his needs in the areas of self-care and physical function, safety, comfort, and social and economic concerns. In order to assist with these areas, the most important consideration is optimal restoration physically. This improves his cosmesis, ability to take care of himself, and ability to hold a meaningful job, which gives status and personal satisfaction, as well as an income. The patient must be taught to substitute secondary life goals relating to his primary needs. This can be done verbally, but is more effectively done by example. The patient should be allowed to demonstrate to himself whether he can or cannot do his previous type of work or how he might do his previous type of work with necessary adaptations. Alternative lines of work may also need to be investigated.

The handedness of an acquired amputee remains the same, although retraining to use the other arm is desirable. The remaining arm becomes much more skillful than it was before and is better than the artificial arm. Most congenital amputees naturally use the normal remaining limb as the dominant extremity, whether it is the upper or the lower limb. I have knowledge of a rare amputee born minus one limb who feels awkward with the limb that is normal and is convinced that her dominance normally would have been on the absent side. Even after half a lifetime using the normal limb, this individual still feels awkward using this limb, despite the fact that she has never worn a functional prosthesis and has never had the experience of having a right upper extremity. An amputee without a right hand has the same difficulties as any left-handed individual and, in addition, has manipulation and prehension only on one side. A person with only one limb obviously is severely disabled if even minor injuries occur to this limb. Many have nightmares about injury or loss of the remaining limb.

Amputees consider themselves less handicapped than normal individuals consider them. They view themselves as essentially normal with minor handicaps irrespective of the severity of their functional loss. They greatly desire to be in closely knit social groups but feel themselves excluded, more frequently with adults than with children. Amputees are reluctant to ask for help unless it is really needed, especially from strangers.

There appears to be a great difference in how often people ask for help (Sharples, 1969). Some people ask for help relatively frequently; the more independent person does not ask often. Some people are very disturbed by having to ask and even more disturbed when unwanted help is offered. People spontaneously offer help, often when it is not a necessity. Most patients accept most of the time: The reason stated for accepting when it is not needed is because the normal individual feels "giving" when helping out a disabled person. Therefore, patients accept, feeling that they are doing the nondisabled individual a favor. In addition, they state that they get tired of rejecting unneeded help, since people resent offering help that is not accepted. There are some amputees who persistently deny even needed aid. Mature patients politely refuse help when it is not needed, but do not make a fuss over it, since they realize that if they refuse aggressively, the person offering may well not aid some other disabled person when that other person requires help.

It has been my experience that the amputee finds great difficulty in discussing amputation, even with those people trying and trained to be of assistance, such as therapists, physicians, and nurses. Amputees sometimes even have difficulty discussing the amputation with other amputees, since some consider this an invasion of privacy. As a defense, most amputees (or other minority groups) refer to other amputees (or members of their group) as "them" and not "us."

Amputees often find thinking about the amputation very painful and, in the attempt to investigate the psychology of the amputee, I have had repeated experiences with amputees who became quite disturbed after some preliminary discussions, because they were brought to think about events and problems that they had pushed into their subconscious. They became more critical and more aware of their problems than they had been prior to the discussions. This is why any survey that investigates an individual's attitudes in one session is bound to be self-limiting. Some amputees in a wheelchair curse the wheelchair, even when they know that it is required for their well-being.

The worst nightmare in the life of any unilateral amputee is the threat of losing the opposite extremity. This is not purely fear of loss of function, but a fear of complete impotence. They often describe waking up at night in drenching sweats because of this nightmare. This occurs not only to vascular and traumatic amputees, but in patients with congenital anomalies as well.

Some amputees resign themselves to the life of a hermit and accomplish nothing. Others, as a compensation for their loss, find it necessary to prove themselves in the real world and become excessively competitive. Others try to accomplish new things as a constant challenge.

For the individuals who have children, more commonly for women than for men, the emotional disability is visible in the children of the amputee, even though the physical disability is not. Children have a great deal of emotional conflict regarding the amputation of their parents' limbs both because of the comments of their playmates and their own distaste. In addition, they occasionally are required to do things for the amputee parent that they would otherwise not have to do.

Amputees are extremely sensitive concerning their disability and feel that they are treated as a separate class of people and not as individuals. Often they feel that they are treated as "things" or ignored or treated as subhuman or asexual. Their sensitivity to society's treatment of them is almost identical to the feelings of other minority groups, whether racial or religious.

Many congenital amputees never having felt the sensation of having all four limbs are curious to know how it would be to have the function, but more important, the sensations of all limbs. They occasionally express jealousy of their spouses for having two limbs. They feel that things are done "effortlessly" by people with all their limbs and feel themselves "inefficient." The traumatic amputee considers himself inferior, which causes feelings of self-doubt and self-pity, often resulting in self-indulgence and the desire for emotional support. Other amputees become responsible and help support people emotionally weaker than themselves. Whether they crack under the additional emotional strain or whether they become stronger because of it depends upon the strength of their character. As with fine china placed in the kiln, disability cracks some individuals, but those who survive the process become stronger than ever.

Traumatic amputees feel that congenital amputees are probably not as conscious of their amputee status as traumatics, since they have never had the part and are not as conscious of the sense of loss. They do not feel as much guilt or as embarrassed. Traumatic amputees, according to their reports, feel much guilt and embarrassment. Congenital amputees feel "defective" and inferior, but not guilty.

A number of amputees have stressed that being made responsible for important tasks is extremely important in instituting the feeling of self-respect. If this is not given, they tend to give up social activities and other challenges. Love and affection are at least as necessary for the disabled as for the normal individual, but this must be expressed in not only giving privileges and benefits, but in insisting on the amputee becoming a responsible member of a closely knit family and community. This applies to both adult and child amputees.

Some people are emotionally destroyed by an amputation, such as the great Cole Porter, who never wrote another hit song after his amputation. It is obvious that his amputation did not affect his ability to write music, except for its emotional impact. Other individuals appear to mature more rapidly and become extremely successful, perhaps more successful than they would otherwise have been after they have been in the crucible of disability and have been able to conquer the fires of misfortune. If the amputation occurs at certain stages in psychosexual development, this may prove to be very detrimental. A teenage amputation is extremely traumatic. Child amputees have times in their lives during which schooling is interrupted or mediocre. They may have great pain, their friends disappear, and they are isolated. Strong father and mother images and strong family ties are very helpful, provided they do not overprotect the individual. The basic personality is not changed if the amputation is above the age of six, but only modified.

Rehabilitation personnel are looked at in many ways by amputees. Except for medical treatment and surgery, doctors and nurses are viewed as being unimportant in the rehabilitation phase of treatment. Physical and occupational therapists and their aides who assist with carry-over appear to be of most significance. Social workers often are felt to be detrimental, as was found by Sharples (1969). Psychologists are viewed as irrelevant. Vocational counseling services are viewed as important but totally inadequate to the needs of most amputees. Many amputees feel that they would have liked to have had contact with other patients and parents once the acute phase of care was over in order to be able to learn from the experience of others.

Social workers are frequently viewed as meddlers who refuse to help with environmental manipulation. Instead, they tend to be interested primarily in the psychological interactions of the family.

The relationships of amputees during the acute and chronic stages of their care appear to depend far less on the medical and paramedical staff than we would like to believe. For most individuals, therapists of the same sex are preferable, except for those individuals who have difficulty relating to their own sex. This depends upon the individual's upbringing and home life, which are crucial. The title and training of members of the medical team are viewed by amputees as almost irrelevant. One of my patients visited the psychologist at least twice a week for two years and yet told me that he never once talked about significant facts to her but saved for her only insignificant and impersonal things, because of a lack of closeness. Most amputees make friends with other patients as individuals at least during the time they are hospitalized. These friendships are occasionally maintained but frequently abandoned if the patients move away. Nurse's aides and therapists are at least as important as physicians in helping a patient over the emotional rough spots during his care. This depends upon the personality of the clinician in relationship to the patient and upon the feeling of true friendship and respect between the two individuals. Most amputees, especially in the acute phase, need to have proved to them that the person trying to help them is a friend. This is usually accomplished by talking as a human being, rather than as a therapist. Most patients judge this by conversation about matters other than the medical care, what most would consider "irrelevant" talk.

An important criterion for some individuals is that the therapist come to see the patient and chat with him on his own time. It must appear to the patient that the therapist goes out of his way to be a friend. Significant individuals for amputees are those that they view as friends, even if the persons are not knowledgeable about the specifics of care for the problems concerned. Patients accept the opinions of untrained or poorly trained people over those of more expert individuals, if they consider the less trained person more a friend.

Success in life as an amputee depends not upon the treatment given, but upon the individual's inner strength. Treatment is primarily providing an environment in which a person with motivation can learn on his own with hints from the therapy staff as to what other amputees have found successful. Early training may not be used immediately if the patient's emotional state does not permit. Early exposure to training and prosthetic use provides the patient with the knowledge that function is possible. If, at a later date, the emotional state changes in such a way that the patient wishes to obtain optimal function, he then either remembers what has been taught or knows where to go. Training thus acts as a base for experimentation and adaptation by a motivated patient. When a patient changes a way of doing something, a therapist should be flattered and gratified. The therapist's function is to provide the foundation upon which the life of the patient is built.

Kessler (1951) considers that an effective counseling tool is the use of other amputees. He writes,

> One of the most effective tools in the armamentarium of the amputee counselor is demonstrations by persons with similar or more severe physical disabilities. Amputees who have made satisfactory adjustments and use their artificial limbs with skill provide a great measure of encouragement to the patient whose rehabilitation is still ahead of him. The competitive spirit is aroused, and the patient feels that if another can do so well, perhaps he can, also. In this connection, the various group demonstrations put on from time to time by successful amputees are immensely reassuring. Some of the artificial limb companies stage annual outings which feature competitive sports events, and occasionally hospitals or civic groups sponsor these demonstrations. Several of these have been conducted by the Office of Vocational Rehabilitation of the Federal Security Agency in cooperation with the American Medical Association and other groups. These demonstrations, called "Amputees in Action," embrace a variety of sport and athletic activities such as skating,

dancing, boxing, bowling, fishing, baseball, gymnastic activities, and badminton, performed by single and double arm and leg amputees.

Taking into account the stresses imposed by limb loss, it is not surprising that sometimes the stress is more than the patient can cope with. Maladjustment may appear in the amputee in many forms: (1) withdrawing, retiring, reticent, isolated behavior; (2) shy, timid, self-conscious, fearful behavior; (3) refusal to recognize the real condition, concealment, and delusions; (4) feelings of inferiority; (5) overly serious, thoughtful behavior; (6) emotional and psychosexual immaturity; (7) asocial behavior; (8) paranoid reactions, sensitivity, and suspiciousness; (9) craving for affection, love of praise, and seeking of attention; (10) excessively high goals; (11) extremely aggressive competitive behavior; and (12) anxiety, nervousness, and temper tantrums.

The nature of the disability is relatively unimportant as far as predicting the quality of the behavior and feelings are concerned. The reactions to permanently disabling injuries change with time. The emotional reactions to complete loss of function are somewhat easier than to partial loss of function, perhaps because dependency is clearly inevitable.

The reactions are aspects of the normal psychic defense reactions. It is very helpful when the patient's reactions are discussed with him openly and frankly. He should be assured that you are not being critical, but have seen the reactions before and understand them. Each reaction has its consequences in the life of the individual. Where they are beneficial, they should be retained. Where they inhibit the person from realizing his goals, he should be asked to consider changing the overt manifestations of his feelings so that they don't impede him.

It may take some time for the person to admit to himself that his ability to cope with his situation can be improved. It is always easier to blame outside forces for one's lack of success. Psychoanalysis may be helpful in this regard.

## Chapter IV

# PROSTHESIS LIMITATIONS AND REJECTION

It is important for the patient and his doctor and family to understand what he can and cannot do with the prosthesis. There is only one way that I know to determine what a patient can do, and that is for him to try. The doctor and the patient can together estimate the patient's functional potential, knowing the components and the patient's abilities and limitations. In order to prescribe adequately for a patient, the doctor must discuss the patient's life goals with him. The patient must work together with the other members of the team to attempt to attain as many of his life goals as are feasible and where it is not feasible, to help the patient to modify those goals.

I have learned through experience that it is usually futile to attempt to tell a patient that he cannot do certain things. I have found a few people who can do almost anything with a prosthesis. I am careful not to be overly optimistic concerning a patient's functional end result, since patients are discouraged when they find that they cannot perform as well as expected.

The amputee who has an amputation because of malignant tumor has, in addition to the general feelings of the amputee, a fear of impending death. In my experience, no matter what has or has not been told to the patient, he suspects that the amputation was done for a malignant tumor and generally fears the worst. Except in rare instances, I have found that an adequate discussion of the patient's problem is the most effective way of getting the patient to cooperate and understand the problems involved. By an adequate discussion, I mean discussion in which the fact of malignancy is confronted and the patient informed that while in every type of malignancy some people die early, many survive for their normal life span.

Average life expectancy is not given, since I point out to the patient that any average is composed of people who do better than average and some who do worse, and I cannot tell at which point on the continuum the particular patient may be. I always attempt to retain optimism as long as possible in the patient. Certain families try to hide the reason for the amputation from the patient. I have found it to be almost uniformly unsuccessful. Certain patients will deny the malignancy even if they have been told of it, and when denial or "disinterest" occurs, I do not press the point, since this defense mechanism is adequate for some individuals. I let the patient ask any questions he wants and answer them honestly. I do not force information on him.

Amputees for peripheral vascular disease generally have forced upon them the necessity for amputation by the progression of their disease. The attempts to save the limb have brought the possibility of amputation home to him, and it is generally easier to explain amputation to this patient. Some resist amputation far beyond reason, and considerable discussion with this patient and with the family is imperative in all these cases.

There is no direct relationship between the extent of the amputation and the psychological problems that occur. This is due to the fact that the psychological problems are more a result of the patient's previous psychological state than they are a result of the functional loss. With amputation, the patient has functional limitations. Whether they interfere with his life-style depends on the life-style. The patient can either circumvent the limitations, avoid them altogether, or attempt to compensate by using remaining facilities or an artificial limb. Any choice involves compromises and an appreciation that only partial satisfaction can be obtained. An amputee may fail because of inadequacies in prosthetic design and fabrication or because he cannot always control the prosthesis adequately. The man-machine interface cannot be designed to be completely reliable in its transfer of information and function in both directions. A failure may thus be in the patient, the prosthesis, or the interaction between the two. The amputee must get accustomed to occasional failure. If his tolerance for failure is limited, this may be a reason for rejecting a prosthesis.

Wilson (1970) wisely points out that the acceptance rate of arm prostheses, both body and externally powered, is very low.

The reason is, "the usefulness of present-day assistance is so marginal that, if the clinic team fails to apply any one part of a system properly, failure of acceptance is likely to result." He declares that, in the upper limb especially, although commonly in the lower limb as well, prostheses are prescribed for the level of amputation, rather than for individual patient need. Fortunately for the leg amputee, the lower-limb prostheses are less marginal than the upper, because of the closer approximation of prosthetic function to normal function than in the upper limb.

Failure also occurs because of discomfort while wearing the prosthesis. One quarter of all amputees of the upper extremity complain about discomfort from the prosthesis. This is one of the most common causes for rejection of an upper-limb prosthesis. Arm amputees are much less tolerant of discomfort than leg amputees, since their function is better with one hand than it would be with one leg. The discomfort is due to abnormally distributed pressures, irritation and discomfort due to heat and perspiration, abnormal sensations, pain, and excessive energy expenditure leading to fatigue.

One aspect of fatigue that is frequently neglected is the psychological fatigue that occurs because the amputee must pay attention to prosthetic usage with nonautomatic feedback mechanisms in addition to paying attention to other aspects of his activity. Whereas the normal individual has a closed-loop sensory feedback mechanism from his joints, tendons, and muscles, the amputee does not have this and, thus, must use secondary information from other sense organs, such as the eyes, to have some appreciation of where his foot or hand is at any given moment. This additional attention that must be paid to what is ordinarily an automatic unconscious act, requires psychic energy to be used, making it unavailable for other matters. While the significance of this factor is hard to assess for any individual, its effect on amputee prosthetic rejection is significant in certain cases.

Amputees experience emotional as well as physical difficulties in wearing prostheses related to excessive perspiration, pain due to neuromata or inadequate prosthetic fit, mechanical failure of the prosthesis, fatigue, difficulties in learning to operate the prostheses, and poor neuromuscular coordination leading to functional difficulties. Mechanical and functional disorders, and secondary medical problems disappear when the problems are solved. The frustration remains. Emotional problems that may interfere with fitting are many and are less amenable to rapid resolution. Some patients expect a prosthesis to feel just like a normal limb. Those that so expect who are not informed to the contrary or who cannot accept it do not tolerate any discomfort and frequently reject the best prosthesis. This occurs commonly in patients who are not informed of the almost universal existence of the phantom-limb sensation. They frequently do not tell the doctor about their concerns that center primarily upon the fear they are emotionally unbalanced. They relate the sensation to a poorly fitting prosthesis.

Patients lacking the motivation to learn to use a prosthesis may use it as long as they are in treatment, but discard the prosthesis on the first available occasion. The occasion usually occurs when some minor factor interferes with prosthetic use, especially when the individual must pay for the repair. The prosthesis then goes into a closet, never to be seen again. One indication of lack of motivation is a patient who says that he wore a prosthesis for some years, but then when it no longer fit or there was some problem with it, he did not return for adjustments or to obtain a new prosthesis. It is my experience that it is useless to prescribe a new prosthesis for this category of patient, since he will, at the first opportunity, again abandon the prosthesis. The time and money used in obtaining a prosthesis and in retraining him in its use are wasted.

The difference between a symptom and a complaint is important in this regard. The patient feels a symptom but complains about it because it is annoying. This depends upon the intensity of the symptom and the patient's ability to tolerate it. The tolerance partly depends upon the emotional significance of the symptom. If the patient feels something which he fears is life-threatening, he may either go to a physician immediately to confirm or deny the frightening possibility or may reject going to a physician, so that he will not hear bad news. Other patients magnify each minor symptom into a major complaint because of their need for dependency, sympathy, and attention. This is an emotional need and is related to prosthetic problems only peripherally. If the patient's prosthesis were perfect, this individual would undoubtedly find another symptom to complain about. Some hysterical manifestations may be treated by hypnotism. The symptom disappears, but the basic emotional problem breaks out in some other way.

There are many individuals who "shop" for doctors, and amputees are no exception. Some amputees go from clinic to clinic and from prosthetist to prosthetist, always seeking something new and better. Some degree of this is desirable for reassurance and optimal care. It can be carried to extremes. Unfortunately, some newer devices are publicized for professional or commercial exploitation, with no real advantages over older equipment. The "shopper" is attracted to such an institution and may spend enormous amounts of time and money for little benefit. These patients are a problem to the profession, since they downgrade the intelligence and ability of each member of all clinics that they have visited prior to the latest one. The most recent clinic can be certain that at the first hint of something new somewhere else, their clinic will be spoken of in the same disparaging light as the previous clinics. It is partly for this reason that it is important to be as honest as one can with amputees, not only about the advantages of artificial limbs but also about the disadvantages. This is especially important in trying sophisticated and expensive research devices.

Not all patients are adept at using mechanical aids. Some people do not have good neuromuscular coordination and have difficulty in learning to use any type of prosthesis because of their awkwardness. They are unhappy, since they see that other amputees function at a much greater skill level than they can. Most often they blame the prosthetist, the doctor, the therapist, or all of them together. A review of the patient's neuromuscular disabilities and past history in sports or dancing, etc., may indicate the real problem. Trying to convince the patient of this may be difficult. Inadequate use of the prosthesis and lack of proper maintenance increases maintenance costs and dissatisfaction.

Anxious individuals appear at the clinic at the slightest suggestion of a change in prosthetic function. This type is a "worrier." Maintenance and clinic costs rise because of the constant presence of these individuals. I have not been successful in managing these people. The opposite extreme is the patient who never comes to the clinic, even when the prosthesis is almost destroyed. He appears long after he should have, stump in terrible condition, and the prosthesis is beyond repair. If he had come in while the problems were minor, the prosthesis possibly could have been salvaged, and a prolonged period of recuperation from stump damage could have been avoided. Prosthesis rejection is rare in this person. Routine rechecks may help, but that keeps people dependent. Dependency is the opposite of rehabilitation.

Conformity with each society's standards of attractiveness is important. This is a problem for all amputees. The abnormalities of gross appearance are of concern to an amputee who is wearing a hook instead of a hand. Less obvious problems, such as abnormalities in gait, noise from prosthetic components, or the click of a hard below-elbow socket on the table or a noisy knee joint, may be disconcerting to other individuals. Unless corrected, these faults are a cause of dismay with the device.

McKenzie (1970) reports difficulties with acceptance of a prosthesis because of lack of cosmesis, both dynamic and static. The cosmetic functional hand is used dynamically in ways that the natural hand is not, and thus, the cosmetic effect is ruined. Excessive motions of the shoulder and elbow to compensate for the limited adaptability of the terminal device for allowing correct approach for prehension ruin the cosmetic illusion, which is good at rest.

There are many amputees who cannot or will not understand the explanations given to them regarding cosmesis and function and the problems involved in prosthetic fitting. There are amputees who, despite many explanations, insist that the prosthesis look exactly like their normal limb. This is despite the fact that it has been explained to them that even normal limbs do not look the same from moment to moment. Some amputees expect that the prosthesis will have no finite thickness or weight, and will be the same size, feel, and shape as their normal limb. To a minor extent, this is a matter of ignorance. More importantly, this is usually a psychic rejection of the prosthesis and the amputation. Unless these patients can be changed in some way, it is almost impossible to train them adequately in the use of a prosthesis and to get them to accept the prosthesis. These patients come back to the clinic with innumerable complaints that can never be resolved. As soon as one complaint is taken care of, another complaint crops up. In some patients, multiple and varying complaints are a daily occurrence. If the prosthesis is adequate, the clinic team can do nothing but inform the patient that there is nothing else that need be done, and he must get accustomed to it. With increasing use of the prosthesis and an improvement in their ability to use it, these patients, on occasion, learn to accept the prosthesis and complain about it less. If this does not occur, the only recourse is referral for psychiatric care. In my experience, this is rarely effective. The educational level of the patient is much less important in this regard than the patient's previous emotional state, except in those patients who are frankly mentally defective.

Any inadequacy in limb design or construction inhibits function. Inadequate fit is surely the most important of these. The patient must learn to control the prosthesis, and because of the nature of the attachment of the prosthesis to the body, truly satisfactory control is impossible to achieve. His training must be such that he has adequate voluntary neuromuscular control to get the prosthesis to function at its optimum. The present state of the art does not permit one to be satisfied with the devices and available techniques. For this reason, the amputee must be taught to anticipate a significant number of instances in which almost normal activity is impossible or at best extremely difficult, especially during the training phase. The training phase not only teaches the patient what he can do with the prosthesis with proper training but also, at the same time, teaches him what cannot be done with a prosthesis.

All prostheses are, to some degree, uncomfortable. What is regarded as a comfortable prosthesis is one with a tolerable degree of discomfort. The patient must be acclimatized to a device that is inherently unstable, restricts perspiration from the stump and irritates the skin, is quite heavy, and does not do all that he wishes it would do. We must, therefore, make every effort to maximize comfort when possible. In addition to the discomfort of the prosthesis, phantom sensation or pain may be annoying and frightening. The patient wearing a prosthesis is subject to higher energy expenditure than the normal individual. This predisposes to fatigue. Part of the energy expenditure is due to the fact that the biomechanical characteristics of the missing limb are nowhere near duplicated in the prosthetic limb. The amputee must pay continuous attention to the control of the prosthesis, using psychological as well as physical energy. All of these stresses take their emotional toll.

After treatment, three quarters of amputees say they feel they have become adapted to the loss of their limbs, while prior to fitting and training, only one third of amputees feel adapted to the loss of a limb (Fishman, 1962). I believe that both figures are very high. Patients deemphasize feelings of inadequacy and loss of body integrity. Almost 90 percent of amputees told Fishman that they rarely if ever feel regret about the loss of their limb. This is in marked contrast to the fact that more than half of amputees have fantasies related to their being two-handed individuals again. What they tell a friend is different from what they tell an unknown interviewer.

The greatest problem in being an upper-limb amputee is the inability to perform at the previous level of activity; another is the loss of cosmesis; and still another is being different from other people. Although more than one half of arm amputees relate their major problem as being due to lack of functional ability, there is little doubt that the majority of amputees are more concerned with appearance and being different from other people. Men in particular do not like to admit that they are concerned over appearance, which is thought to be a female trait.

The ability to accept the loss of an arm depends on the amputee's conscious and unconscious interpretation of his status. Factors relating to nonacceptance of amputee status are fear of reduction in functional potential, of reduced sexual potency, that amputation has relegated him to an inferior social status, and of vocational difficulties. Those people who were seeking means of escaping from competition and had a desire for dependency accept the amputee state well, although many feel the need to put on a facade of dissatisfaction. Real acceptance of amputation, if it exists, depends upon the awareness of the individual that he can work toward overcoming part of the disability to achieve his maximal potential.

Although most amputees profit psychologically as well as functionally from the use of a prosthesis, there are a significant number of amputees who do not, as pointed out by Fishman (1962). The reasons for unsatisfactory prosthetic adjustment appear to be:

> (a) . . . very little information concerning prostheses is available to new amputees early in the rehabilitation program and this deficiency encourages the development of unrealistic expectations concerning prosthetic wear.
> (b) Overly optimistic anticipations concerning the value of prostheses were, in most cases, modified downward after prosthetic wear and were accompanied by considerable personal disappointment and stress.
> (c) No attempt is ordinarily made to alter pessimistic attitudes towards prosthetic wear prior to fitting.

While Fishman feels that "on the basis of these findings one might conclude that it is not appropriate to provide a prosthetic appliance to an individual until he has developed an attitudinal predisposition to accept its purposes and functions," it is my experience that the provision of a prosthesis immediately after amputation or very shortly thereafter has a positive educational value for the patient. It appears to me that prolonged delay prior to fitting a prosthesis predisposes to the reinforcement of negative attitudes toward the amputee status and prostheses. For some individuals, prosthesis use decreases their function. For them, rejection of prostheses should be viewed as a positive development.

People react to the world in ways reflecting their perception of the world and not necessarily reality. For that reason, at the same time the patient's physical and functional losses are being worked upon, it is important to have his perceptions of new status reflect reality as accurately as possible. While this occasionally needs formalized psychotherapeutic treatment, the difficulties inherent during an active rehabilitation program in the presence of other amputees reinforce the perception of reality.

Weiss et al. (1971) found a consistent relationship between motivation as measured by the absence of personality encapsulation and constriction and better self-related prosthetic adjustment. They found that sociopathic impulsivity, as reflected in colliding or invading figures on the Bender-Gestalt Test were significantly related to self-rated prosthetic adjustment. An amputee's impulsive behavior on this test was related to lesser satisfaction with prosthetic restoration and, to some degree, with tampering with the prosthesis.

The Weiss group (1971) reports that lack of certain feelings about the values of prosthetic rehabilitation appears related to dissatisfaction with prosthetic wear.

Weiss et al. (1971) found that below-knee amputees adjusted consistently better than above-knee amputees. Below-knee amputees had better self-ratings and professional ratings. The prosthetists rated the patients most favorably, the physicians and therapists intermediate, and the vocational counselors rated the patients least favorably.

The measures of surface pain and deep-pressure sensitivity were significantly related to the self-rating criteria. Those patients who are most sensitive to deep pain had generally poor prosthetic acceptance. Tactile sensation was less well correlated. Weiss et al. (1971) found that freedom from phantom limb pain gave better adjustment, mainly among below-knee amputees. With advancing age came decreasing success and self-rating.

Sensory feedback is extremely important. It exists to a minor degree through the harness and socket of prostheses, especially in patients who have had amputations early in life. Weinstein (1968) has shown that there is a progressive increase in sensitivity in the skin of the proximal stump subsequent to amputation.

## Chapter V

# THE LIMB-DEFICIENT CHILD

THE CONGENITAL AMPUTEE presents another emotional picture entirely. The child has no emotional problems relating to the fact of being an amputee, except those transmitted to him by his parents and other members of society. The parents ordinarily have feelings of guilt and inadequacy. The congenital amputee is not aware of any abnormality until he can appreciate differences between people and the difference is called to his attention. Children between the ages of three and five need reassurance and an explanation of the cause of the amputation. It is about that age that they become significantly aware of differences in people. Congenital amputees take a long time to adjust to the fact that they are different. Congenital amputees have difficulty in remembering when they first realized that they were different from other individuals. This, to a great extent, depends on the home life and the stress that the parents placed on the difference. It is my experience that patients start to realize that they are different from other children between two and three years of age. The children sometimes feel guilt over "evil thoughts," such as death wishes towards parents and siblings, and traumatic amputation may be viewed as punishment for those thoughts.

Kinnier-Wilson (1970) points out the many personal losses that children with reduction deformities face. There is a loss of image, not only of body but image in function. There are differences in temperament, due to difficulties the severely disabled have in adjusting to their loss. The motor loss is great, due to muscle weakness, joint inefficiency, and lever arm shortening, implying loss of reach. In addition, if such a patient wears a prosthesis, he has a loss of stability at the junction between the socket and his stump, inadequate force, loss of range of motion at the articulations, inability to perform some movements, unnatural arm patterns, lack of coordination in function-oriented movement, inability to vary the motion of the prosthesis to within as great a range as the human arm in prehension force and size, adaptability to shape, fine manipulation and positioning, and sensory transduction for temperature, texture, contact, vibration, pain, and light and deep touch.

In addition to the loss in mobility, strength, and ability to manipulate finely, the control system, cosmesis, and sensory input are all markedly reduced. As Marquardt (1969) has so ably pointed out, learning and understanding are markedly impaired, unless sensory stimulation occurs. A child cannot learn the nature of surfaces, weight, size, and resilience, unless the appropriate sensation is stimulated early enough. He may not appreciate the fact that the constituents of an object may not be uniform throughout the object. Stereognosis or the shape of specific objects may not be fully understood without appreciation of its form by the sense of touch. There is not only a problem with the body-prosthesis interface, but also a problem at the prosthesis-task interface. Kinnier-Wilson (1970) writes, "The child without specific sensory training is learning about the world through tongs, so to speak. In other words, the prosthesis isolates the child from the world through its own specific stereotype of movement and its barrier to sensation."

The congenital amputee wonders what it would be like to have the limb that he is missing. He has never known what it is to have it, and therefore, is probably less affected by the absence than patients who have an acquired amputation. The girl with bilateral congenital absence of both arms and congenital leg absence mentioned previously, appears to be more disabled by the loss of both arms than by the absence of one leg. Despite this, she feels that she would want a leg more than an arm, although cosmetically and functionally, she would be better off with one or both arms. She would prefer a leg not just for walking but for running, skating, and skiing, both on snow and on water, etc. These are things that she has never been able to do, while she can do many things with her artificial arms.

Most amputees feel that patients with acquired amputations, either due to trauma or disease, feel the same sense of loss, while congenital limb-deficient persons really do not miss the limbs but wonder how it would be to have them. Comparison of individual reactions is not possible, unless a limb-deficient person who subsequently loses another limb is discovered. One man with whom I came in contact related no significant differences in emotional response.

Patients who have had an amputation for a very long time use their prostheses as part of their body. They may joke about the prosthesis and often refer to their hooks as "my hands." They use them, to some extent, as organs of expression, shrugging the prosthetic shoulder or pointing with the prosthesis for emphasis. Occasionally, patients with bilateral hooks caress a loved one with the hook. Some normal individuals hold hands with a bilateral upper-limb amputee by holding the hook and feeling perfectly natural doing it. An arm amputee can hold a loved one in an embrace and enjoys the body contact where such is possible.

Most amputees feel that attending school with normal children is much better for an amputee than attending a school for the orthopedically handicapped. Where this is possible, I would agree that this is desirable. In general, physical treatment time should not be taken from time needed for schooling, since this inhibits the learning process. Medical treatment, if elective, should be after school or during school holidays.

For the teenager who becomes an amputee because of a malignant tumor, the fear of death hovers over and complicates the reactions to becoming an amputee. Teenagers who are amputees because of trauma may feel guilt because they participated in the causation of the amputation. There is always the fear for the future, and the uncertainty of how it will affect their lives educationally, economically, maritally, vocationally, and in terms of hobbies and sports.

### Family Attitudes

Giving birth to a disabled child is a great emotional shock. This is especially true with respect to a limb-deficient child, since the disability is obvious. While the emotional reactions are experienced by both parents, the mother is most affected. Suicide is frequent, as is psychotic breakdown. This generally occurs a few months after the child is born. A woman who has given birth to a congenital amputee is generally overridden with guilt, because of some real or imagined sin for which she is being punished by having a disabled child. There are feelings of inferiority and a sense of failure as a person in having given birth to a defective individual. She is afraid of having defective genes and chromosomes or attempts to find out if any one is defective in her own or her marital partner's family tree to apportion blame. Often the spouse is blamed as a failure as a person and as having defective genes. There is a sense of both guilt and pity, and this vacillates as a cycle.

The reactions to the birth of a disabled child may be rejection, excessive coddling, or alternation of both. The birth of a congenital amputee to a young couple without other children may be devastating and is a frequent cause of divorce. Frequently, the parents do not have another child. A search for drug causes may be undertaken, with lawsuits being fairly frequent against drug companies and physicians.

When the child is emotionally rejected, he may be physically as well as emotionally abandoned or abused. The child may be kept hidden from society. Even in large cities with well-developed medical services, deformed children are frequently not seen in an amputee clinic for a long period because of parental shame. Extreme attempts to hide the amputation may be made. When the children are eventually seen, the prime goal of the parents is cosmesis, in an attempt to hide the existence of amputation. Infanticide is not uncommon.

The mother's reactions, of course, reflect onto the child. Her distaste gives rise to the child's self-hate. Later reactions of other individuals affect the personality of a child, but none so much as the above-mentioned feelings of the mother. Mothers, even in our society, frequently, consciously or unconsciously, get rid of their abnormal children either by killing, abandoning, or ignoring them. As compensation for these feelings, many mothers overprotect their children. The parents must be encouraged to speak freely about their feelings and fears. Mentioning that these are expected is of help.

The child with a congenital amputation is generally spoiled

and not disciplined. This lack of discipline creates sibling jealousy. Often, the siblings are spanked after some mischief has been done, even when the deformed child is the guilty person. Sibling jealousy arises from the extra care and time spent with, and lack of punishment of, the amputee. The amputee is, of course, jealous of his normal siblings for their ability to perform better than he can. Frequently, it is important to teach the amputee one or more skills at which he can best his normal siblings. Teaching him a sport, such as horseback riding or use of a trampoline, may be helpful. He should be taught to excel in at least one thing, while the other children dissipate their energies and skills among many different activities. This is crucial in the development of his feelings of self-worth.

Many congenital amputees have few, if any, friends until they go to school. The entire family of a woman who has given birth to a congenital amputee may be considered inadequate. Neighboring parents may forbid their child to play with the amputee, as if the deformation were contagious. This is, to a great extent, the basis for the killing of deformed children at birth in many societies, including the present. The feelings of the mother are reflected in the feelings of inferiority of the congenital amputee.

Society considers the amputee inferior not only physically, but in every other sense. This is the internalized self-concept against which the successful amputee wages an incessant fight, frequently leading to overcompensation. Some of these patients as adults remember that they asked their parents when their limb will finish growing. At about five, the impact of their amputation appears to strike them most strongly. Some congenital female amputees who grow up to have children are even more terrified of having a disabled child than the normal woman. A number of congenital amputees who eventually gave birth to normal children confess to seriously considering suicide prenatally if their children had been born abnormal. This is despite the fact that their own adjustment in life would generally be considered as good.

The parents may feel guilt and that the child's abnormality is a punishment for sin. It is odd that some atheists feel the same way. The parents blame themselves and each other, and the grandparents blame the in-laws. These children frequently make poor adjustments in later life not because of the functional insufficiency, but because of the psychic abnormalities fostered in them. The overprotectiveness of parents is frequently interspersed with reminders to the child of how inconvenient it is for the parents to have a disabled child and how the life of the parent or sibling is modified adversely by the very existence of the child. These children, on the one hand, feel rejected and, at the same time, overprotected. It is very important to emphasize to the parents and grandparents early the importance of treating the child as nearly normally as possible, including assigning chores and administering appropriate punishment to the child. Family groups of parents of limb deficient children are extremely helpful in aiding families to cope with the emotional, social, economic, educational and nurturing problems they encounter.

Because of the primitive fear of genetic transmission of disability, amputees may have difficulty with potential or actual mates and in-laws. In our society, it is still remarkably common to expect that amputation in a parent can be passed on to the child. While less common, this fear exists even for traumatic amputations. Many people are incapable of relating to disabled people, and family conflicts are frequent after amputation, as with other disabling conditions. Many persons do not relate well to amputees and tend to shun their company in social as well as in employment situations. It is not only strangers and employers, but also fellow employees and family who tend to look on the amputee as an object of pity and occasionally of distaste. The amputee looks at himself in the same way. He soon learns to anticipate rejection from others and, in fact, may find it where it does not exist. This sensitivity is common to all disabled persons and is a reaction very similar to those found in other minority groups.

Both sexes find that the amputation may cause family disruption. Many mates leave their spouses after the spouse has an amputation. Probably more men leave women when the woman has an amputation than vice versa, since physical attractiveness is a more important criterion in judging women than men in our culture.

Patients who have an acquired amputation often fear that their children may be born with defects and want to see their children immediately to make sure that they are normal. Even sophisticated people fear that their own disabilities may be transmitted, even when their disabilities were not congenital. This may inhibit both sex and procreation.

Males have a great fear of loss of sexual potency after their amputation. They not only feel a sense of loss but literally feel castrated. Impotence is frequent. Compensatory satyriasis and infidelity may occur.

For long-term progress in minimizing the psychic consequences of the disabled, one must reduce the internalized antipathy of society. That can only be done by getting society to accept the disabled. The reduction of the isolation of the disabled requires, for children, *mainstreaming* in school so that normal children have frequent contact with those less fortunate than they are. This makes the amputee less frightening in school, on the playground, and later at the work bench.

## Chapter VI

# SOCIAL ASPECTS OF REHABILITATION

THE EMOTIONAL EFFECTS of amputation are often a social and vocational problem, not only because of the functional loss imposed by the amputation but primarily because of the obviousness of the defect. One congenital bilateral above-elbow and unilateral hip-disarticulation amputee had exactly the same degree of emotional and social reactions as a congenital amputee with only a partial hand amputation. The reason is that the minor upper-extremity defect was almost as obvious as the major limb absences. Thus, a patient with a facial scar has a severe psychological, social, and vocational handicap, irrespective of the fact that functionally he has absolutely no loss. This has been shown in some studies of criminals with facial disfigurement. After plastic surgery removed a part of their disfigurement, a greater percentage were rehabilitatable. A person with a moderately severe functional loss, such as an above-knee amputee, may have few psychological and social problems, provided his gait is cosmetic. Lower-limb amputees have a lesser problem than arm amputees, because their defects are less obvious.

Reactions are very individual. Most amputees prefer to think of themselves as normal individuals and, therefore, look for their friends and acquaintances among nondisabled people. This is especially true among those who have been raised among nonhandicapped people. Dating reactions are very individual and depend as much on the patient as upon the person of the opposite sex. Some individuals are repulsed by stumps, deformed limbs, or prostheses, while others take them naturally. Still others have sex fetishes concerning stumps and/or prostheses and seek out amputees as mates and sexual partners. Groups of persons who now seek sex with amputees are in existence. (*Penthouse:* Forum, 1972, 1973; Wolff, 1977; "Stud With a Stump," 1977).

Few people admit their distaste at seeing the disabled; it is socially gauche. The distaste is manifested in many different ways. It may be, for example by avoidance, oversolicitousness, pity, superstition, or fear. The reactions to the amputee may be any or all of these. These emotions are not confined to the superstitious and ignorant, but are found in all of us. As an example, one of the people whom I wished to engage to edit my books could not begin to edit the chapter on the history of amputation. In declining to do the work, she wrote, "To admit the truth, it was not only lack of ability, but partly also revulsion that blocked my progress." This intelligent and fine woman found that she could not even work on editing a chapter on amputation history. You can imagine the difficulty she might have had attempting to work on sections dealing with surgery or congenital amputation.

It is the emotional attitudes that are such an impeding factor in the total rehabilitation of the amputee. These feelings are kept hidden when possible, but they burst forth during a challenge, such as when an amputee applies for a job or asks for a date. I know of one square dance stopped in the middle when a man refused to take, as a temporary dance partner, a woman with a congenital hand defect.

Every amputee knows that these feelings exist in the minds and hearts of others because he himself has harbored the same emotions and thoughts. One of the greatest blocks to understanding, the only path to rehabilitation, is to deny that these problem feelings exist and therefore to do nothing to correct them.

The amputee has many experiences with nondisabled individuals to whom he must become accustomed and learn to react appropriately. The nondisabled show curiosity, pity, and sympathy and tend to isolate the amputee. Able-bodied individuals expect that the disabled have a second-rate life-style. The nonhandicapped are frequently surprised and sometimes resentful if the disabled are demonstrated to live a first-rate life-style. Nondisabled individuals expect the disabled to withdraw from contact with normal individuals and to seclude themselves.

People stare at the amputee, attempt to help when help is not needed, and treat him differently. Social participation is frequently diminished. Amputees wish to keep their disability private, because it reminds them that they are different. Whether the amputee is ashamed of this disability or not determines how he relates to the outside world's staring and questioning. If he rejects the disability and himself, he resists offers of help and expressions of pity. Amputees consider staring as much more of an intrusion into their personal lives than a direct question. It may be because staring is a more impersonal act. Amputees react differently depending upon when people stare at them, depending upon mood and the actions of the individual doing the staring. All amputees are aware that people look at them on the street and elsewhere. Generally, they object to this feeling but if the staring is unobtrusive, they usually let it pass. If the staring is obvious, frequently the only reaction and probably the best one is for the amputee to give the individual a "dirty look." Occasionally, amputees make remarks under these conditions, but most realize that if they pick a fight with such an individual, they are handicapped in such an encounter and might get hurt. Even if the ensuing altercation is merely verbal, amputees are generally aware that a normal individual can say a number of things very painful to hear. Altercations, even verbal, are therefore studiously avoided. Hostility is internalized.

When amputees are asked questions about their amputation, they resent it, depending upon who is doing the asking and the way the questions are phrased. If someone they know well asks a question, they generally answer appropriately and in as much detail as they wish to give. When relative strangers ask questions, amputees generally do not resent it too much, provided the question is only "Were you born that way?" or "Was it due to an accident?" It is strangers asking detailed questions who are most resented. The questions appear to be frequent.

Amputees object to questions more from adults than from children. Most amputees, especially of the upper limb, say that they are stared at almost every day, especially when they use public transportation. When a child is around an amputee, he is generally fascinated by both the amputation stump and the artificial limb. He generally will try to feel it and ask questions about it. Even when questions are not asked, they very often try surreptitiously to feel it to try to understand. This occurs even after years of contact with a family member with an amputation.

The discussion of amputation is less traumatic when it is done by the therapeutic staff or by close friends or family. Many amputees wish to appear psychologically well-adjusted and, therefore, resist talking about their disability. The need for self-esteem is great, and reassurance that the amputee is a valuable person in the eyes of the amputee clinic staff and others is important. It is frequently helpful to point out that a person's basic difference from other animals and all other people resides in his mind and in his "heart."

The valuable distinctly human characteristics of thought, concern, and caring for others are not affected by amputation. Patients cope with psychological assaults on them by various means. The patient may become aggressive and verbally attack the person who noticed the amputation. This may take many forms. One way of coping with disability is to avoid all reference to it. The disability may also be minimized, in order to preserve a relationship. One can do this by redirecting the conversation when it treads on dangerous ground, that is, speaking superficially about the subject. In essence, this is a tactic of withdrawal from a dangerous psychological situation. The problem of children who notice and comment upon disability is well known. Children with their frankness, sometimes innocent and sometimes not, can wound the amputee deeply, especially when the amputee assumes that his amputation is not noticed. The child's comment upon it brings to the fore all of the previously repressed emotions and fears.

White, Wright, and Dembo (1948) declare that amputees prefer that outside individuals:

(1) not discuss the amputation unless the amputee brings up the subject;
(2) not ask questions immediately;
(3) take into account the amputee's mood;
(4) not persist in discussing the subject if the amputee is not de-

sirous of doing so. If the amputee wishes to discuss the amputation, the nonamputee should not try to change the subject.

The amputee makes new friends readily if he is young, although it is harder than for the nondisabled. The new friends are made wherever the child may be, as with any youngster. The older amputee has greater difficulty in making new friends and tries to retain the old. Even with old friends, new relationships emerge, so the old friends must be treated as new.

One of the things that a normal individual resents most is a disabled person attempting to give advice to him, since the normal thinks the disabled person inferior in all respects. This attitude has been reported to me by many amputees and people with other handicaps. This makes it almost certain that handicapped persons rarely rise to managerial positions for which they may otherwise be qualified.

Since a limp is more common and acceptable than the sight of an artificial limb, lower-limb amputees have somewhat less difficulty in social acceptance than upper-limb amputees, provided the public does not know that the person is wearing an artificial limb. A limp may be caused by temporary injury or disease, both of which are more acceptable than amputation. Attention may be paid to the amputee upon seeing the prosthesis or hearing mechanical noises. Noises may be useful to assist function, but are detrimental in regard to social acceptance.

The reaction of individuals to the sight of an amputation stump in a patient not wearing a prosthesis or the sight of a prosthesis, varies with the individual and his experience with disabled individuals, especially amputees, but also may vary dependent upon the person's sex, age, the time of the day, the distance of the individual from the amputee, or the individual's preoccupation with something else. For example, a problem in traveling found by many amputees, especially of the upper limb, is when they arrive at a hotel at night and the hotel desk clerk is not very busy. The sight of the prosthesis or of the stump generally shocks these individuals, especially if they are somewhat drowsy and sleepy. Their reactions may vary from staring to close to a faint. The same desk clerk seeing the amputee during the day when many people are about generally has a much lesser reaction.

The reaction of most individuals is shock, bewilderment, and distaste. This is reduced by a cosmetic hand, but some amputees feel that a cosmetic hand is "a lie" and that they must face up to being amputees. The amputee is extremely sensitive to other people's reactions. The amputee appears to become more rather than less sensitive with time, in many cases. Most amputees find that very little sympathy is given to their amputee status, except by rare individuals.

After being an amputee for a long period of time, frequently an amputee will repress his knowledge of the emotional reactions of other people. Amputees avoid the staring and questions by conscious and unconscious tricks, such as keeping the amputated hand in the pocket, going always to the same stores and using the same buses each day, so that new people will not be met. By always riding the same bus, they are assured that the same people will be riding with them each day, so that the strangeness wears off and they will be stared at less. On entering a subway car, many stay near the door they enter and hide the prosthesis or stump in or behind their clothing, a newspaper, or a book. They try not to walk through the bus or train, so as to avoid attracting attention.

Amputees try to avoid meeting new people more than the average. Many amputees find that other people never forget them or their names. Amputees with average memories often forget other people's names, as do we all. This may be embarrassing, since other people remember the amputee because he has a characteristic that stands out, while to the amputee, there is nothing particularly outstanding about the nonamputee. Some amputees feel the need to show their amputation to strangers on first meeting them. This is to "declare oneself." If the person reacts adversely, no relationship can be established. If, on the other hand, there is less adverse reaction, then the individual feels that a relationship can be established, and efforts will be made to establish one.

An important concept pointed out by Siller and Silverman (1958) is that there are many considerations important when any person attempts to assess the appearance of a prosthesis. He first relates to the appearance in static situations. The second relates to the naturalness of movement and use, or the dynamic appearance. An additional factor is the intimacy of contact between the amputee and the observer, the factor that Siller and Silverman call the *intensity* of the situation. This depends upon the closeness of the relationship between the observer and the amputee and the attention that the observer focuses upon the situation. If the observer is distracted by other events, then the prosthesis may not register upon his consciousness. When distractions are few, and the observer has little else to distract his attention or the prosthesis is obvious, then the appearance is noted. One of the tricks used by amputees to reduce the obviousness of the defect is to use eye-catching mechanisms. Female leg amputees may wear bright hats and facial makeup to distract the eyes from the lower limbs. Arm amputees may use eye makeup, hats, or daring skirts to distract attention from the upper limbs. The key to a person's reaction is the obviousness of the defect.

Young children are very inquisitive. They invariably ask questions in a rather natural manner and when answered, adapt to the individual's status as an amputee and then forget the amputation. Some children are shy and do not ask questions, but if they are told about the amputation, it generally stops mattering. As the child grows to teenage, he is more aware of the amputation and is generally somewhat more shy about asking than the younger children. Adults demonstrate much more distaste by their facial expression than do teenagers, who in turn express more distaste than young children.

Only 2 percent of Siller and Silverman's (1958) group felt that people were always looking at them. All my arm amputees are concerned about this problem. I have yet to meet an upper-limb amputee in whom this is not the most serious problem that he faces. Amputees take considerable pains to avoid being conspicuous, even when only part of one finger is lost. This depends upon the obviousness of the loss. Even a patient with a minor loss often keeps the limb in the pocket, hides the prosthesis behind his back, and refuses to cross the length of a bus or subway car. In Siller and Silverman's group, 67 percent denied feeling resentment of curiosity of other people. I have yet to find a single individual who denies this resentment once he respects and trusts the doctor-questioner. This is irrespective of whether the amputation was congenital, traumatic, or due to disease. I agree with Siller and Silverman (1958) when they say that what amputees describe as acceptance of their disability by the public is in actuality a wish fulfillment more than a reality. They ascribe to normal individuals attitudes that they wish society had to them, rather than acknowledge that society looks upon the amputee at best with indifference and at worst with active distaste.

Most amputees look for nonamputee mates and friends. They try not to consider their disability as very important and relate to themselves as normal. They prefer to avoid the company of disabled people. They reject the handicapped label and other handicapped individuals, especially individuals with an obvious physical defect. Some able-bodied individuals look for amputated patients as mates, since this makes them feel relatively stronger. There is a cult of men who have sexual fetishes of amputation stumps and/or artificial limbs (*Penthouse:* Forum). Pointing up this fact to a recent female amputee may be reassuring, but is not always welcome news.

Most if not all amputees express their inferiority feelings only to other amputees and not to able-bodied individuals. This is why amputee clubs are so valuable. To normal individuals, the amputee almost always relates that he feels as if he were almost normal or normal. This feeling of inferiority probably is greater among males than females. Men seem to need more reassurance of their sexual prowess and ability to cope with the world than women do; perhaps they bear greater responsibilities in a family. Women tolerate cosmetic loss poorly; appearance is of very great importance to their self-esteem.

In the relations between the sexes, there is considerable difference. A young male traumatic amputee does not feel particularly insecure with boys, provided he can compete with them. An upper-limb amputee can fight very well with his hooks, so he feels almost equal to his fellows, except in those activities in which he cannot participate. This appears to be because status among boys is, to a great extent, determined by the ability to fight. A male traumatic amputee, however, feels insecure among girls. This is normal during the teens even among the nondisabled. The cosmetic loss is important to girls. Girls feel inferior in competition with other girls for male company. This sense of inferiority with the opposite sex is extremely important. Some amputees date anyone of the opposite sex who will go out with them. This is one factor in the exploitation sexually of the disabled by other disabled individuals and by normals. Many girls use sexual promiscuity and/or drugs to attract male companionship. The novelty value of having sex with a disabled person appears to be very attractive to some individuals. For the insecure nonamputee, it may be the only time he is potent. In relation to the opposite sex, it appears that whether one person or the other is exploited depends primarily upon the relative malleability of one individual and the manipulative ability of the other. Some amputees manipulate other individuals, but are not themselves manipulated, while others are easily manipulated and exploited, economically, socially, and sexually. This appears to depend upon the individual's initial personality far more than it does upon any formal training or subsequent experience.

Amputees of either sex are often used by physically normal individuals as sexual objects, since the nonphysically handicapped individual is aware that the amputee has difficulty in social relationships far in excess of the nonamputee. They thus become easy prey for individuals seeking purely physical relationships. In the sexual sphere, there are many physically normal individuals who are insecure emotionally—emotionally disabled. They may have feelings of inferiority and impotence with physically normal individuals. They may feel dependent and weak, except in the presence of the disabled, to whom they can feel superior and in relation to whom they are relied upon. For this individual, sexual relationships and indeed marriage provide them with the strength to enter other competitive situations.

Patients with severe physical disability are often married to physically normal individuals, often therapists and nurses. Therapists relate very well to the disabled and find it easy to justify marriage to severely handicapped persons as an act of liberalism or charity. As a matter of fact, frequently this is to compensate for their own emotional disabilities. A great number of physically normal individuals, who are impotent with the normal, find themselves potent with the amputee. The amputee in his relationships sometimes can take advantage of this weakness in the physically normal individual in a number of other ways, since the sexual potency of the physically intact person depends upon the acquiescence and cooperation of the amputee. It is not to be thought that this type of reaction is one-sided, however. The amputee in turn exploits physically intact individuals. Many amputees perfectly capable of doing activities with relative ease exploit the pity and guilt of other individuals by obtaining favors, such as special consideration on public vehicles or lower prices for certain purchases or helping with activities of daily living and on the job. On some occasions, a person will do a job perfectly well by himself when there is no one to exploit, but will act helpless so as to get help on those days when it is available.

In relation to the opposite sex, in addition to the insecurity and inferiority feelings mentioned previously, the realistic lack of ability to live a full life in all senses for those with multiple limb loss may impinge upon the relationship. Very important emotional relationships and interactions may exist, rarely elicited from patients because of their personal nature. One upper-limb bilateral amputee mentioned to me that the major disappointment of his girl friend was that he could not express sentiment and affection manually. This boy is not spontaneously verbal. In addition to this, the normal caressing activities cannot be done adequately to suit his girl friend. One of his disappointments is that he cannot run his fingers through her hair. This is of emotional importance to her. He has two hooks. When it was mentioned to him that he could rest his cheek on her hair as a symbol of affection, he pointed out that this had a different emotional connotation both to him and to her. Communication by caressing and gesticulation is important, and deprivation of these functions may lead to feelings of social isolation. Most congenital amputees using prostheses do caress and gesticulate with their terminal devices after prolonged wear.

Amputees appear to favor as mates physically intact individuals. If they marry or date disabled individuals, they prefer them to have different disabilities, so that their functions are complementary and they can help each other with various functional needs. A bilateral arm amputee, for example, would probably not date or marry another bilateral arm amputee, because neither one could help the other with significant activities.

Amputees feel that girls and women are more cosmetic conscious and that the absence of an arm is especially important. Generally, girls are still more passive in meeting people, especially men, and therefore, are afraid of not being approached. This passivity is now decreasing. Male amputees can approach a woman, who may refuse, but they have the freedom to do the approaching. It is felt by amputees that this is easier. Limb loss in a male is a problem, because he is looked on as the protector and provider for a family, which requires greater strength and endurance.

Some amputees state that they would not marry another disabled person, since they feel that they could not take care of their own problems and assist someone else who also has problems. This appears to be a dependency wish; to have someone help them with their problems, but to be unwilling or unable to help a mate with their problems.

In this regard, amputees assume that the nondisabled individual has no problems that the amputee can help them solve. This is the attitude of the nondisabled also. A few secure amputees seek dependent mates. Marriage for amputees is possible even subsequent to their amputation. Unmarried women have as their greatest fear that they will not be able to marry. This is a significant problem. Most female amputees overcompensate and use their personalities to attract prospective husbands. This is wise. It is helpful for the amputee to have someone with whom to discuss this problem, especially someone who had an amputation and subsequently got married. The amputee club needs this kind of participation. Most women amputees prefer to start off on an "honest" basis, so when they meet a date, they inform him very early that they have a defect, so that whatever emotional responses may occur happen before deep emotional involvement sets in.

Amputation early in life tends to leave emotional residuals of dependency, hypochondriasis, and other emotional concomitants. There are a great number of individuals who find satisfaction in having a dependent spouse. I find that some individuals apparently seek out the disabled and weak as marriage mates. These marriages tend to be stable. However, if amputation occurs after marriage, especially amputation of an upper limb, this is not infrequently a cause for divorce.

Men treat the marriageable woman amputee in one of a number of ways. The first is to treat her as a "rare bird" and to become interested in her because of her amputation. Men generally probe her to see whether she is really "human." They then begin to feel somewhat more comfortable with her and to deal with her more as a normal individual. The second and more frequent way of meeting the problem is for the man to be shocked and, therefore, to retreat. The woman amputee is therefore ignored, and no significant contact is possible. Most women amputees feel that it takes a male longer to forget their disability than it takes other women. This may be because of the interactions expected in persons of opposite sexes. Some women amputees have few male friends, and those who have, find most of the friendships superficial. Social contacts are a problem, and time is needed by the amputee to adjust to the problem. Most women amputees find they must be more outgoing than most women, which, with the changes in our society, is becoming easier. Some men date a woman amputee to show that they are "liberal." Other males assume that a woman amputee is easy sexual prey, and thus seek out women amputees and other women with disabilities. Insecure men feel more able to dominate an amputee. The fetish cult has been mentioned.

Women amputees, especially of the upper limb, consider other women who try to mother them obnoxious. Sports-minded women often do not give the amputee a chance to get close, since many of them wrongly consider the amputee, especially of the upper extremity, as incapable of participating in any sports, and therefore incorrectly assume that they have no common interests. Women interested in home and family have a somewhat better reaction, since they may have certain things to discuss with the woman amputee. If the woman amputee is unmarried, however, they may consider her pitiable and unable to compete for a husband.

There is a considerable amount of exploitation of and by the amputee. This exploitation takes place in many spheres in life. Normal individuals exploit the disabled and amputees in particular by hiring them for jobs at a lower salary level than they hire the nondisabled. The reason for this is that the amputee has difficulty in obtaining a job, and thus takes any job, even though it is at a lower pay scale than what a normal individual could obtain under the same circumstances. Promotions to a higher grade are slower. While many real estate agents and owners of apartment buildings will not rent or sell homes to the disabled, some of those who do, do so at higher prices.

Amputees often tend to take advantage of pity and occasionally not only use their amputated state for begging for their own benefit, but allow themselves to be used by others for collecting money for charitable causes. When they collect money for charity, they often bring in far greater amounts of money than the able-bodied. Some severely disabled individuals feel that the only exploitation to which they have been subjected has been by medical personnel who have used them for teaching purposes and publicity. This certainly exists. The limbless person should get something out of the relationship as a *quid pro quo*.

With the disabled, as with the able-bodied individual, good looks, a smile, and a pleasing personality go a long way in seducing others to grant advantages they would not ordinarily grant. For the amputee, this may be of special importance. Fear of embarrassment is occasionally used as a weapon to obtain services and help. Each amputee must be made aware of his or her individual advantages and disadvantages and of the methods most appropriate in specific circumstances.

As with most minority groups, the amputee is not above taking advantage of someone with a similar disability. The values of society in general are present in the amputee. Members of minority groups tend to assume the values of the majority group. An amputee with a lesser disability thus often feels himself superior to an amputee more disabled, emotionally or physically. Thus, persons with a disability exploit other persons with disabilities when they can, in exactly the same way as a nondisabled person exploits an amputee. Thus, an amputee with a below-knee amputation, for example, may well exploit, sexually, or otherwise, a person of the opposite sex having multiple anomalies or amputations or a person with a different disability. The amputee has identical emotional characteristics to the nonamputee. The vices and virtues and strengths and weaknesses of each are identical. The interreaction of these factors makes a fascinating study.

Most amputees feel that regular schooling and jobs are frightening at the beginning. Leaving the protective environment of the hospital or rehabilitation center early is of great importance, since it forces the individual to face the real rather than a protective world. Most hospitals and rehabilitation centers are correctly viewed by amputees as being entirely too protective. Most amputees who eventually become successful in their adjustments state that some means of decreasing the protectiveness in the hospital and in the outpatient clinic is needed to slowly wean the patient away from the protective environment and those in the therapeutic team who would overprotect them. Most patients feel that, while weekends at home are a small step in this direction, additional measures are needed. The reason for this is that their friends have other commitments. Often, the amputee feels that he is imposing if he calls up and ties up a day or evening with a former friend. These friends appear to forget the patient and become involved in other things. Patients generally spend the entire weekend at home with the family or friends, without meeting strangers who have not seen their amputation before. They do not make an opportunity to go shopping and endure the stares and attention of others. The medical personnel are viewed as overprotective, and special efforts need to be made to compensate for this. Patients often unconsciously avoid being seen by strangers.

The medical-social worker should be primarily of help in environmental manipulation, assisting the patient in getting help from appropriate social agencies to pay for the cost of hospitalization, obtaining the prosthesis and learning its use, and in referral to appropriate sources of vocational education and training. Housing and transportation may be crucial concerns, as is some method of income maintenance while the patient cannot work. Homemaking services may be needed. Architectural changes in the home may be desirable as ordered by the doctor, after evaluation and consultation with the physical and occupational therapists, and may be obtained through various social agencies through the help of the social worker. The social worker also has the responsibility for planning care after discharge and referral to a nursing home, where this is indicated.

The medical-social worker also has the responsibility of a social casework interview and an evaluation of the patient, including his social and psychological background, adjustment to amputation, and feelings regarding the use of a prosthesis. The medical-social worker's evaluation, along with that of the psychologist and psychiatrist, if necessary, helps to analyze the patient's psychological strengths and weaknesses and the resources s/he has to deal with stress. While most medical-social workers prefer those aspects of their work dealing with the last-named functions, in my view and in the view of most amputees, they are most helpful when dealing with the environmental-manipulation aspects of their functions.

The psychological consequences of having an obvious disability reflect not only the patient's sense of loss and shame, but also society's evaluation of what disability is and acceptance of disabled individuals. Unfortunately, society still all too often wrongly considers the amputee a useless cripple. In order to change society's pressures on the individual, a public-education program is needed, starting very early in elementary school, so that the disabled person is accepted as an otherwise normal person, rather than as someone apart. It is for this reason that where amputee children can compete effectively in public schools they should be allowed and encouraged to do so. This requires the education of school principals and teachers who frequently keep these patients out of their regular classrooms because of the teacher's psychological sets. The excuses used range from the ordinary to rather elaborate excuses. One excuse often heard is that the lower-limb amputee "could not run out of the building fast enough in case of fire." It is not true.

Every amputee can and should engage in gymnasium activities, sports, extracurricular activities, and otherwise participate in the social life of the school, both during and after school hours. While it requires some imagination on the part of the teachers to modify the program to suit the needs of the child, this is required if any meaningful dent is to be made in public attitudes toward the amputee. Unless we are willing to work on these attitudes, the traditional isolation and segregation of the amputee will continue. The amputee must not be allowed to continue to be thought of as a creature apart from normal human existence. Education is needed, more of the nondisabled than of the disabled child. This allows the future growth of social and recreational, as well as vocational, interaction between the able-bodied population and the amputee.

When a patient has undergone an amputation, it is important that close contacts be maintained between the patient's family and community. There is a great tendency toward physically and emotionally abandoning the amputee to the care of the hospital and nursing home, psychologically cutting him off from the possibility of returning to a full social and industrial existence outside of the hospital setting. In order to avoid the abandonment of the patient to the therapeutic team, the problems of the patient must be kept in the forefront of the minds of the family, employer, and friends. This may be done by involving the community in the life of the amputee and the amputee in community life. The concept of the *therapeutic community* used in psychiatric institutions and in rehabilitation is a helpful first step toward this goal.

We must concentrate attention on the paradoxical problems of patient motivation. These are reflected with all of the disabled. They relate to the need to remain a member of his family and vocational communities, despite the fear of rejection and failure. In addition, the secondary gains of disability, both economic and dependency, may prove formidable stumbling blocks.

The utilization for the amputee of the day-care principle as used for the mentally ill may prove of value. In this method of treatment, patients come in for their therapy programs during the day, frequently on an all-day basis, but go home for the evening and to sleep. This involves the patient in family activities and vice versa. One problem with day-care centers for amputees is transportation. Transportation costs are high. However, hospitalization costs are much higher. Another problem is that most rehabilitation facilities do not have adequate space or personnel to be able to accommodate a large number of amputees in all-day therapy. Even when patients are in a rehabilitation center, they frequently spend at most two or three hours in therapy daily, and the rest of the time is spent watching television and in diversional, recreational situations. Recreational diversions used in a therapeutic manner are desirable. There is a tendency for the recreational aspects to be emphasized and the therapeutic aspects of recreation minimized. Therapeutic recreation needs to be made more therapeutic with more personnel trained in group physical and social interaction, with specific training and expertise in order to fulfill truly its function of encouraging the patient to participate in community activities, both within and outside of the treatment setting.

The therapeutic community must truly involve the community and not only within the hospital. It cannot be taken as a matter of course that the patient will be accepted back into the family and to the world of work without a conscious desire and effort to educate the family and community. Education of the family is probably best done through self-help clubs and group therapy sessions, in which the patients and their families can freely express their needs, desires, and fears to each other, so that they can work out their mutual problems together. This requires a skilled group therapist who can unobtrusively lead the fearful patient and his family into productive group discussions. In this way, patients and their families can discuss home modifications, attitudes about disability, the problems of work, fears of sexual inadequacy, difficulties with change in living situations, and economics, etc. It avoids the all-too-common criticism of therapeutic personnel by the amputee and his family, "What do you know about the problem, you still have both legs?"

The lack of adequate follow-up of amputees is widespread. I have seen amputees who have not had their prostheses checked in more than twenty years. With present communication and education this problem is slowly diminishing, at least in the large urban centers; the problem, however, remains acute in rural areas and in the smaller urban areas, and particularly so for the poorly educated and the socially deprived. The above relates to the immediate care of the patient's prosthesis and his stump. It can safely be said that adequate follow-up of the patient's needs in areas other than the strictly surgical and prosthetic are almost nonexistent anywhere in the United States. There are almost no programs attempting to follow up the patients' social integration, vocational problems, and avocational needs adequately. While it is well known that most amputees can play table tennis, ski, swim, and engage in other sports, how many centers are there that have set up follow-up clinics inquiring of the patient sports activities that would interest him? How many amputee clinics assure that the vocational problems of the amputee are handled optimally? Even the "good" amputee clinics generally are satisfied with referring the patient to the overloaded state divisions of vocational rehabilitation. This serves to "pass the buck" and ease the conscience of the members of the rehabilitation services, but unfortunately in many cases, does not adequately meet the patient's needs. I regretfully admit that circumstances often force me to be equally remiss.

Rehabilitating or reintegrating the amputee into society is the ultimate goal of all treatment. One of the finest expositions of rehabilitation that outlines the principal assumptions and principles of rehabilitation is to be found in *Psychology and Rehabilitation* (1959) by Beatrice A. Wright. She affirms the following:

> The human being is a being of worth to be respected and cherished no matter how severe his disabilities may be. He has a right to be assisted in the unfolding of his personality and in the development of his potentialities for his own sake and for the good of society. The very nature of life implies physical and mental variations. Persons with a disability . . . should partake of the activities that society has to offer. Separation is indicated only under the considered evaluation of personal and social welfare and then only as a temporary expedient until reabsorption into the community at large is possible. Acceptance on the part of society rather than aversion and fear gives the emotional attitude towards which the rehabilitation effort is directed. Although man is beset with physical and mental attributes which often interfere with his well-being, he also has . . . assets which can be supported and developed. . . . Unless special care is taken, being sensitized to the pathogenic can leave one inadequately sensitized to stabilizing and maturity-inducing factors.
>
> Difficulties in employment, cultural attitudes and prejudices, conditions of the physical environment are examples of reality factors with which the person with a disability must cope. . . . The importance of "treating the person as a whole" becomes less of a cliche when it is realized that such areas are interdependent. . . . The patient must assume to the degree feasible an active role in both the planning and executing of his rehabilitation program. Among the foremost consequences are the restoring, maintaining and enhancing the person's initiative and self-respect. . . . Society is obliged to establish schools, hospitals, recreational facilities and work opportunities that will meet the needs of all its members. Where special needs are evident, special arrangements to accommodate them are indicated. . . . Rehabilitation is a continuing process that applies to the individual so long as he needs help and to society as long as conditions exist that interfere with the welfare of any group of its citizens. . . . The process of rehabilitation is complex, it must be subject to constant reexamination.

The problems of severely handicapped amputees are much different than the problems of simple unilateral upper- or lower-extremity amputees, especially in the young. A patient with one amputation below the knee or elbow may have some difficulty in society and in work, but the difficulties relate far more to the individual's personality than to any real functional loss. On the other hand, multiply amputated individuals or amputees with additional medical conditions, such as deafness, blindness, or brain damage, have very severe problems. The multiple amputee, either traumatic or congenital, usually suffers from a severe lack of socialization, since he has difficulty participating in the sports and recreation life of his peers. He tends to be left out of social occasions, in most instances, unless he is a very strong personality. Integration in normal school life and social activity after school is rare. This makes the multiply handicapped person an isolate in most cases.

Part of the isolation comes from overprotection from the family, rejection by school and playmates, fear, and feelings of inferiority of the amputee himself. Because of the lack of integration into life during and after school, children with multiple handicaps are isolated, except from their families. Even those individuals who join a group of disabled youngsters find their ability to socialize is also limited, since most of their day is used for therapy. Their feelings of insecurity and inferiority are marked, especially as it relates to relations with the opposite sex. Girls have a greater problem in this regard than boys, since the worth of a girl in our society is more often considered in terms of her physical attributes than on her ability to function. Reactions depend greatly upon the patient's personality. Some multiply handicapped patients react by becoming aggressive. Others integrate fairly well into society. Most do poorly and retreat into a sheltered, isolated homelife in front of a television set.

It is interesting that, in contrast to the findings of Sharples (1969), most of my amputees found no significant difference in value between the terms *amputee, handicapped,* and *disabled.* The term *cripple,* however, is looked on by almost all as being an insult.

The desire of the disabled to relate their goals and aspirations to the normal population is great. As the severity of the loss increases, it becomes more and more difficult for the amputee to consider himself normal, because of his functional loss. The physical, economic, vocational, and psychological cost to amputees is great for them to be able to attempt to function competitively with those without a handicap. Many will not or cannot pay the price.

## Vocational Considerations

The acceptability of any employee is a complex of many factors, such as his intellect, social status, income, as well as skills and weaknesses. Amputation is a threat to all individuals, not only socially but economically. It is less of a threat for people in professional and executive positions. The greatest threat is to those who use their bodies for a livelihood, such as patients in the low socioeconomic levels and people performing sports and in some of the arts for a living. The poorly educated individual who becomes an amputee frequently remains unemployed. A person has only two things in life to sell to a prospective employer: the work of his brain and/or body. Because the amputee has diminished physical work ability, he must use intellect more than his body. It is for this reason that the amputee population generally has a slightly higher educational level than the able-bodied in the same socioeconomic group if the amputation occurred during early life. There is a great tendency to acquire an education to attempt to compete in the job market. It is a realistic appraisal of salable skills.

Norman Berger (1958) surveyed a large sample of upper-limb amputees. There was a shift from manual work after arm amputation. In the sample, 65 percent were employed in skilled, semiskilled, or unskilled occupations prior to amputation. Only 27 percent remained in that category after amputation. While only 14 percent of the sample engaged in professional, executive, and service occupations before amputation, 41 percent did this type of work after upper-limb amputation. Unemployed individuals were nineteen times as great after amputation.

For lower-limb amputees, the trend was in the same direction, but not as severe, since leg ablation is functionally less damaging than arm amputation.

In vocational rehabilitation of the amputee, thought must be given to the patient's previous skills and the demands of his previous job, in order to avoid later frustration and resentment. Obviously, a person who worked in a sedentary job has less difficulty than a manual laborer. The type of prosthesis must be suitable to the patient's work. Furthermore, the prosthesis must be designed and fabricated in such a reliable way that the patient does not lose an inordinate amount of time from his job because of breakdown of the prosthesis or his stump. The less trouble the patient experiences with the artificial limb, the fewer emotional problems he will exhibit and the better will be his societal reintegration. At the earliest possible time, it is advisable to refer the patient to the state division of vocational rehabilitation for payment for the limb, vocational evaluation, and possible retraining, if the patient cannot go back to his original job. The job title is inadequate to determine whether the patient can go back to his job. Each job, even with the same title, has slight variations in what needs to be done. Only a job-sample technique of evaluation permits a patient to try himself out on a job.

If the amputation requires job change even after training, there are adjustments that must be made in the family and limitations in the patient's view of himself. If the patient starts a new type of job, this often pays less than his previous position. In addition, since he starts on a new job, all seniority in his old place of employment will be lost, there is none in the new, and, as such, economic, status, and emotional consequences are suffered. The managerial and professional person who becomes an amputee seems to suffer less from these losses than patients who are semi- or unskilled. While the psychological consequences of the amputation itself may be similar, the socioeconomic consequences are much greater, the lower the person is on the socioeconomic scale. Because this part of the United States population is the majority, these problems loom large for any amputee clinic team. Selective placement may be needed, or special arrangements may be needed for work. If this is not done, many of these people are unemployable, involving a whole interplay of socioeconomic and psychological problems. A man who was previously economically self-sufficient and respected in the community may thus become an economic ward of the state with a very severe loss in self-esteem because he is on welfare and added to that, loss implied by the amputation.

In order to make the proper decisions, the doctor must truly understand the patient's fears and aspirations, potentialities, and deficiencies. He must also understand the stigma of disability inhibiting the patient's opportunities for employment, even if he has the education and experience otherwise needed.

Frequently, the medical staff acts as if it assumes that the rest of society accepts the disabled on an equal basis with nonimpaired individuals. This error costs the patient dearly. To be considered an equal, an amputee must be better than his competition. The goal of upbringing and rehabilitation must be to strengthen the patient's ability to cope with his problems and to instill in him the knowledge that his work must be superior to that of his competitors both in quality and quantity. His attendance and punctuality and personal characteristics must also be superior to theirs.

Frequently, recommendations are made for the patient to obtain an education to enable him to become a member of one of the professions. In most cases this is sensible advice, but not in all. I know of two cases in which a recommendation was made to attend law school. In one case, the patient has neither arms nor legs. One must question this recommendation, since the patient not only cannot be expected to plead a case in court but, in fact, cannot even be a law clerk since he cannot get the books for himself nor turn the pages to look up precedent cases. Tragic results may occur from this type of recommendation. I have knowledge of a number of cases for whom similar recommendations were made. Subsequently, the patient could not utilize the training which he had worked so diligently to obtain and committed suicide. The suicide rate among the disabled is very high, but the incidence cannot be determined precisely because the suicide is usually hidden. Many of the "accidents" that permeate the lives of amputees are not fortuitous, but are self-inflicted. It is important to warn patients and their parents of these difficulties, so that they may learn to deal with them realistically. We do patients and society a disservice by attempting to hide the difficulties that these patients encounter. I do not mean to imply that severely disabled individuals should not be encouraged to try to succeed in bettering themselves, but only that the difficulties need to be mentioned. Every effort should be made to encourage the handicapped to knock down the barriers that impede their functioning at the highest level possible for them.

Most amputees who hold jobs do so where there is little or no contact with customers, since employers who are willing to hire the handicapped are more apt to do so if they feel that their business will not be damaged because of other people's prejudice against the handicapped. Some employers hire the handicapped only to sell their products, but not for manufacturing or office personnel, so they can advertise that they employ the handicapped.

### Legal Impediments to Rehabilitation

Some of the adverse factors in psychological restoration of the patient to accepting himself as a worthy member of society relate to the financial aspects of workmen's compensation statutes and the laws on liability. If a patient lost his limb through accident rather than through a disease process, our laws as presently constituted tend to work against rehabilitation. There is a seeming financial advantage to maintaining the disability in most workmen's compensation and liability suits. Because of both ignorance and financial gain, some poorly informed attorneys encourage continued disability on the part of the patient so that the patient receives a greater monetary award. The factors usually ignored include the fact that the patient would probably be better off receiving a lesser settlement and earning more. The monetary "advantage" to the amputee serves to encourage maximal disability and minimal functional recovery both on the conscious and unconscious levels. Often, it is not the attorney who brings this to the fore but misinterpretation on the part of family and friends of the patient. If there is no detailed discussion and illustration of the total economic consequences, this may prove disastrous to any meaningful rehabilitation program.

These factors are added to the psychological stress factors of amputation and rehabilitation in general.

### Therapy Staff Inhibition of Rehabilitation

The members of the therapeutic team may unconsciously inhibit true rehabilitation. This may occur because the therapist needs to feel needed and, thus, encourages continued patient dependence.

The goal of rehabilitation is complete patient independence. This means we should aim for the time when there is no longer need to "follow" the patient, as he is independent, and we do not need him. We should refer to the man who does not come for routine appointments as "rehabilitated" and not "uncooperative."

The amputee must be taught how to take care of himself and when to seek our help. After that, he should be left alone to live his life as he sees fit, without our meddling.

Chapter VII

# THE PHANTOM-LIMB PHENOMENON

THE LOSS OF A PART of the body is frequently associated with the feeling that the cut off part of the body is still there. This is referred to as *phantom sensation*. It is a hard-to-define sensation of the presence of the amputated part. This may be an awareness of the presence of the limb or might progress to a faint, pleasant, tingling sensation. The phantom sensation is usually not unpleasant. It can, however, occasionally give itching or tingling feelings. These may occur with weather changes.

The sensation of phantom limb was first recorded by Ambroise Paré (1551). It has been reported by Weinstein et al. (1964) that the phantom phenomenon occurs not only in amputation of a limb, but also in numerous other conditions, such as breast amputation, cosmetic surgery of the nose and other parts of the body, and tooth extraction. It has even been reported that one of the causes of recurrence of weight gain after weight loss by obese patients is their phantom sensation and body image of themselves as obese persons. Sensitive, intelligent, and neurotic individuals are more prone to phantom sensation and phantom pain than less imaginative and more emotionally balanced individuals.

The phantom may be so real that people still feel the amputated part able to move. On occasion, a person will get out of bed expecting the amputated leg to bear weight. Many patients continue to have painful corns on the amputated foot. One patient said that the chilblains that he got in the winter of 1914 to 1915 continued to cause pain in his phantom foot. A captain in the R.A.M.C. continued to suffer from tennis elbow in the phantom arm (The Star, 1924). Another report relates how a veteran of World War I, who had his right hand shot off in Flanders, was standing at the curb of a sidewalk and saw a child run in front of a moving automobile. The ex-soldier ran after the child and, as he believed, reached out to snatch her out of the path of danger. All that he had left was the stump of an arm. In his excitement, he experienced the sensation of still owning a right hand, and but for this, the child might have been saved from injury. Instead, believing that he was seizing the child with fingers he no longer had, he went through the motion mentally of grasping her with the phantom hand. All that he actually did was move the stump of his arm. Many such cases are known.

There are many instances of people who have lost limbs who insist upon burial ceremonies for the amputated members and who subsequently have sensations of pain they blame on events happening to the amputated part, such as dampness of the graves, etc.

The phantom-limb phenomenon may stay the same length and intensity for prolonged periods after amputation. Some amputees report that the phantom-limb phenomenon tends to become less and less predominant, but remains the normal length, until it eventually disappears, returning in intensity and in awareness only under special conditions of stress, either emotional or physical, with the use of certain chemical agents, or trauma.

Patients may have phantom sensation continuously, intermittently, or it may be entirely absent. It may gradually disappear. Many writers report that a phantom sensation is experienced more often by arm than leg amputees (Browder and Gallagher, 1948).

When the basic phantom or *basic phantom-limb percept* is absent, the patient can sometimes call up a phantom actively (1) by concentrating on it, (2) by trying to carry out movements in it, (3) by voluntary contraction of the stump musculature, or (4) by voluntary contraction of the musculature of the contralateral limb. Some patients have a spontaneous phantom-limb percept and others only when they think of it. Crönholm (1951) points out that this is true of the normal limb as well. Most people do not perceive their real limbs unless attention is called to it. The basic phantom is continuous and unchanged in some cases and in others is intermittent.

Crönholm (1951) differs from other investigators in finding

that there is no significant difference between arm and leg amputees as regards presence of a basic phantom sensation. He finds that a basic phantom is present significantly more often in proximal than in distal amputees. Crönholm states (1951) that a phantom is more often experienced by older patients a short time after amputation. The extent of the phantom sensation varies in every case and in the same patient on different occasions. When the basic phantom is present, and only certain parts are present, other parts can also be perceived by concentrating on them or by trying to perform movements with them. Many patients claim to feel an entire limb as a phantom but when pressed reveal that they only sense parts of the limbs. Distal parts are usually represented in the phantom, but proximal parts are represented less often. The clarity of the basic phantom may vary from very clear to very vague and indistinct. Clarity varies with stimulation, concentration on the phantom, movement of the phantom, and various stimuli.

Livingston (1945) says that the phantom limb is not a total reproduction of the amputated extremity and that certain parts of the upper limb, such as the wrist, dorsum of the hand, forearm, and upper arm, are rarely perceived. Many patients give the impression that they "feel the whole thing," but on careful examination, it is evident that the presence of much of the phantom limb is inferred from small portions of the hand, foot, or digits. In neither upper nor lower limb does the pattern correspond to the major peripheral nerve distribution. The neuroma is not established early enough to be the determining factor in the initial onset of phantom, since the phantom exists immediately after amputation. Palpation of neuromas causes an electriclike sensation such as "striking your funny bone." In no case does stimulation of a neuroma excite or stimulate typical phantom sensation.

The parts felt most commonly are generally those with the greatest representation in the sensory cerebral cortex. The thumb and the great toe are felt more vividly than the remaining digits. The balls of the digits are felt more than the digital remaining parts. The articulations are felt more vividly than the intervening parts, and the more distal parts are felt more prominently than the proximal.

The phantom-limb phenomenon is useful in certain instances, since it may assist in adaptation to and use of an artificial limb. It can be detrimental, since on occasion, a patient has injured himself by attempting to walk on a limb no longer attached to his body, e.g. when he woke up at night and attempted to go to the toilet while still groggy. Patients have been known to become anxious and even to commit suicide because they thought that they were insane, feeling the presence of a limb which they saw was no longer present. For this reason, its expected occurrence should be mentioned to each patient prior to surgery.

Crönholm (1951) discusses the length of the phantom, i.e. the length of the most distal part of the phantom from the apex of the stump. He found some patients with normal or foreshortened phantoms, but no "extended" phantoms. Other authors use the term *extended phantoms* to mean phantoms in which the sensation is outside the stump. It is not used in this context by Crönholm. Crönholm states that the stump percept varies considerably from case to case. When the phantom is very clear, the patient often has no percept of the stump: The percept is directly continued into the phantom. When the phantom is absent and in some other cases, the patient may experience a stump percept equivalent in shape to the physical stump or different from it. The basic phantom is more often normal in length in lower- than in upper-limb amputees. There seems to be no difference in length percept between proximal and distal amputees. The volume of the phantom has no relation to proximal or distal amputation nor to upper- or lower-limb amputees. This is contrasted with the differences found in percept of length and is different from the impression of Browder and Gallagher (1948). The basic phantom generally has the same shape as the real limb, but is often less differentiated and less detailed than the percept from within a real, healthy limb.

Haber (1956) reports that phantoms are almost universal in adults. The predominant description is that of a mild tingling or certain tightness. None of these cases referred to their phantom limbs as natural; they all reported the characteristic quality of "pins and needles" and tingling. After removal of the extremity, the size and shape of the phantoms were rarely identical with those of a normal limb. There were fading and "dropping-out" of certain parts of the phantoms. Unequal fading was usual. There are reports of voluntary motion in phantom limbs. Persistence of particular preamputation sensations occurred. Some patients had additional features to the phantom, such as rings or wrist watches. In the upper-limb amputee, the phantoms did not seem to change with the presence or absence of prostheses. In lower-limb amputees, the prostheses often fused with the phantom. Often, the phantom became the same length as the normal limb when a prosthesis was worn.

If the phantom fades, proximal portions vanish first, then intervening areas, and finally distal parts (Haber, 1956). The distal regions are felt most vividly even soon after the amputation. Joints are present more than intervening areas. The upper arm is almost never present, the forearm rarely, but the elbow is sometimes present. The rank order of parts corresponds closely to the size of the cortical representation allotted to those parts. The ability to "move" phantom parts fades much more quickly than the ability to experience those parts. Of his amputees, 88 percent could recall phantom sensations at will.

Flexor movements are easier to make than extensor movements in the phantom. Patients whose terminal parts were telescoped into the stump claimed that they could not penetrate solid matter with their phantoms (Haber, 1958). By contrast, 50 percent of those who had extended phantoms, i.e. phantom parts outside of the stump) reported that they could move the phantom through solid objects. In the 50 percent of those with extended phantoms who reported that they could not move their phantoms through solid objects, the extended phantom temporarily disappeared whenever the stump was moved close to some solid object. Many patients attempt to catch a ball with the phantom or perform some other task with it. Phantoms, under certain conditions, may change positions whether they are extended or telescoped.

The threshold to sensation is much lower in the stump than in the homologous part of the intact limb for light touch, two-point discrimination, and point localization (Haber, 1955). The stump therefore becomes much more sensitive and approximates the fingers more than the same part on the contralateral limb in sensitivity. Shrinkage, folding, or stretching of the skin of the stump do not appear to influence the increased stump sensitivity to light touch, two-point discrimination, and point localization. Sensitivity is better on the stumps of men with telescoped than in those reporting extended phantoms. There is no significant relationship between the wearing of an artificial limb and the dimensions, quality, or vividness of the phantom, according to Haber (1955).

Sensations assigned to the phantom can be elicited in amputees by stimulating the stump or other body parts in various ways. They may have a quality similar to the stimulus, or may be abnormal in quality and/or location. They may be spread or restricted. The stimuli may be touch, pinprick, deep pressure, temperature change, micturition, defecation, sexual intercourse, coughing, gasping, drinking hot or cold drinks, or having a full bladder, etc. Henderson and Smyth (1948) state that 90 percent of leg amputees have brief sensations in the phantom or amputation stump at the start of micturition. One half of all lower-limb amputees experience similar sensations on defecation. This is more common in above- than below-knee amputees.

Crönholm (1951) states that reflex sensations in a phantom can be more often elicited when a basic phantom sensation is present to start with and only in those who can stimulate one. He interprets this to mean that a connection must exist between the experience of the phantom and the change in the central nervous system functions. A volley of centripetal impulses in nerves other than those severed at the amputation is integrated in such a way that a sensation assigned to the phantom is experienced. There appears to be no connection between the possibility of eliciting reflex sensations in the phantom and the clarity of the basic phantom, the occurrence or intensity of abnormal sensations in the phantom, the patient's ability to carry out voluntary movements in the phantom, between upper- and lower-limb, proximal and distal amputees, or the interval between amputation and examination. If reflex sensations in the phantom cannot be elicited by pressure on neuromas, they cannot be elicited by touch, pain, or deep pressure on other tissues.

With stimulation, there may be a difference in the quality of the normally localized stimulus and the reflex sensation in the phantom. This is most striking with touch stimuli, but may be clear with others as well. According to Crönholm (1951), the length of the phantom is usually not affected by stimulation of the stump or other body parts by touch, pain, or deep pressure. He did have one exception when a phantom arm of normal length was experienced, if the stimuli were applied to the amputation scar. Reflex stimuli in the phantom were elicited simultaneously in that case. Crönholm points out that stimulation of the stump evokes sensations as if the phantom were physical reality and were itself stimulated.

The stump takes over the sensory functions of the lost limb, especially the hand. It is not due to a central state of hyperexcitability, but to a shift in the central state of functional organization caused by the amputation.

Crönholm (1951) states that, in some cases, increased normally localized stimulus sensitivity on the stump indicates a central state of hyperexcitability in amputees, in conjunction with a shift in the state of functional organization. Increased central nervous system hyperexcitability may be demonstrated by the hyperactivity of proximal musculature, increased pilomotor activity, and increased sweating.

Crönholm (1951) asserts that, in certain cases, the phantom becomes less clear or the abnormal sensations less intense or even extinguished as a result of the stimuli of touch, pain, or deep pressure.

Crönholm avers that grasping the end of the stump firmly seems to diminish the experience of the phantom, possibly because stimulation makes the stump percept more apparent. Touch over small areas does not heighten the experience of the stump percept to the same degree.

The sensation of a phantom limb is frequently diminished while wearing a prosthesis. The use of an elastic stump shrinker, a total-contact socket, or a snug Ace® bandage frequently relieves annoying phantom sensation at night. Some patients squeeze their stumps to rid themselves of phantom pain and phantom sensation. Gillis (1957) believes that this is a form of sensory stimulation that restores "temporarily the balance of the impulses which impinge on a sensorium and so relieve the pain." The increased sensory input increases the central excitatory state of the central nervous system and restores balanced sensory input from the two sides in a unilateral amputee. On occasion, a socket worn at night may prove of benefit for these patients.

Crönholm (1951) is able to elicit sensations of temperature, both normal and abnormal, from a phantom by applying stimuli to the stump.

Crönholm (1951) reports that one quarter of amputees have sensations in their phantoms on urination or defecation. Amputees of the thigh have the most, below-knee patients have fewer, and very few amputees of the upper arm report that they have such sensations. They are generally regarded as unpleasant and abnormal.

He reports that changes in the phantom occur when a patient wears a prosthesis. It may become either clearer or less distinct.

Crönholm (1951) did not find any case where the patient had the illusion of working with a phantom hand while using a prosthesis, although Pitres in 1887 reported that a phantom foot can feel wet if a patient treads in water with his prosthesis, and the patient can feel pain in a phantom when he makes a false step or walks on sharp stones with his prosthesis. Bornstein (1949) mentioned that patients find it particularly difficult to walk with a prosthesis if the phantom leg is flexed at the knee. Henderson and Smyth (1948) found that, almost without exception, the phantom is never felt while wearing the prosthesis but often reappears when it is removed.

Crönholm (1951) avers that the existence of a phantom is independent of whether a patient wears a prosthesis or not. Sometimes, walking in the prosthesis as well as wearing is necessary for extinguishing the phantom. In some patients, the phantom is called up when the patient dons the prosthesis, but vanishes when he walks with it. He found that, in above-knee amputees, the localization of the phantom foot depended upon whether they stood or sat. It is not influenced if one moves the prosthetic knee passively. Thus, if one passively extends the knee of an above-knee artificial limb, the foot of the phantom stays on the floor if the patient is seated. In upper-arm amputees, he found the position and posture of the phantom totally independent of the prosthesis. He states that the posture of the peripheral parts of the phantom could usually be clearly distinguished. The posture usually depended upon the movement the patient tried to perform and was more distinct in arm than in leg amputees.

Crönholm asserts that the phantom usually but not always follows movements in the stump. If the posture of the phantom knee alters when the patient sits up from a lying position, the patient experiences no movement in it, but the posture of the phantom leg is changed. Both the phantom hand and foot take up a posture corresponding to the habitual posture of these members at rest. Sometimes the phantom hand is tightly clenched. In exceptional cases, the fingers are hyperextended. The phantom toes are, in exceptional cases, flexed. He had no case in which the toes were hyperextended.

Crönholm (1951) states that, in one third of his cases, the phantom was localized outside the stump percept and distal to the apex of the stump, i.e. the phantom hand was situated on the line extending the stump percept. In all the other cases, the position of the phantom hand relative to the stump percept was as if a phantom elbow were bent, whether the elbow was experienced or not. In above-knee amputees, Crönholm asserts that, in almost all cases, the phantom foot is localized on the line extending the stump percept when the patient lay down. In all but one of the cases questioned who had above-knee amputations, when they sat up, the phantom foot was in the same position relative to the stump as would have been the real foot if the phantom knee were bent. In one case, the phantom foot remained extending straight out from the stump. In most distal amputees, when the patient moved his stump, the position of the phantom relative to the stump remained unchanged. In proximal amputees, far greater fluctuations occurred. In cases where the phantom sensation was localized inside the stump or at the apex, the position of the phantom remained unchanged relative to the stump percept. In the cases with clear localization outside the stump percept, 67 percent maintained a constant position relative to the stump, in 25 percent it altered, and in one case the position of the phantom became very indistinct. In above-knee amputees, the position of the phantom relative to the stump remained unchanged or became extinguished in a few cases. In most of the cases, when a patient lay still, the phantom was clearly situated distal to the apex of the stump. When the stump was flexed, the phantom leg was stretched at the knee, and the phantom foot was situated in a direct line with the stump percept. In some cases, the phantom knee percept, whether perceived or not, appeared to be bending, and the phantom foot slid proximally along the bed, parallel to the contralateral leg. In one case, the phantom became localized inside the stump on flexion of the stump even though it was outside it ordinarily.

Crönholm (1951) states that almost all patients could move the phantom, and in these cases, muscular contractions of the stump could be noted in almost all. The contractions are generally throughout the entire stump and seem to be poorly differentiated. There is a difference between the flexors and extensors, each group being more active in the appropriate movement of the phantom. Sometimes these movements are so minor that the patient may not notice them. Movement in the contralateral limb can facilitate or hinder phantom movements.

The phantom is aligned with the stump and moves with it. When the stump is brought near the patient's body or an external object, the phantom often seems to pass through the object without arousing the feeling of obstruction. Weiss et al. (1971) says that the phantom is never felt as an exact replica of the amputated part. Upper-limb phantoms are considerably stronger and more enduring than those of the lower limb. Voluntary motion is frequent, especially in the upper limbs. The nonexistent fingers can be moved through flexion and extension, with flexion more common than extension. Abduction and adduction are usually lost. The higher the level of amputation, the more restricted the impression of voluntary motion in a nonexistent digit becomes. The length of the phantom may be changed by immersion of the stump or of the contralateral limb in warm or cold water, by procaine hydrochloride injection, ethyl chloride spray, application of weights to the stump, and with changing body posture.

Some patients progressively lose their phantom pain and sensation. Frequently stretching the amputated part of the extremity gives relief, in addition to rubbing or scratching the end of the stump. The phantom sensation is peculiar in other ways. For example, if the phantom knee is flexed, when the patient lies on his stomach on the bed, the phantom foot and lower leg appear to stick up through the bedclothes. When the patient turns, the phantom limb turns also but when the patient lies on his back or sits in bed flexing the phantom knee, the phantom limb does not seem to go down through the mattress. A pinching sensation is frequent.

Kallio (1952) studied a group of hand amputees who had been subjected to Krukenberg operations. In this procedure, the radius is separated from the ulna. The phantom sensation, in these cases, felt as if the hand were split, with the radial fingers acting as a unit and the ring and little fingers acting as another. Kallio considered this as proof in favor of the peripheral-causation against the central theory, because such an unnatural hand could never have been part of the body image. There are many reports attempting to show that the phantom sensation may have origins which are central, peripheral, or a combination of both. In addition, there are those who insist that it is of psychogenic origin.

Crönholm (1951) found that the experience of patients with phantoms, walking with a prosthesis, fell into four groups. Some patients have *phantom gait;* they experience a phantom and a more or less clear illustion of walking on it. Pressure on the phantom foot is felt when placing the foot of the prosthesis on the ground. The pressure usually is less clear than on the non-amputated side. The second group has a *vague phantom gait;* this phantom usually follows the posture and movement of the prosthesis, but there is no clear illustion of "using" the phantom, nor is there an experience of clearly walking with the phantom attached to the stump. The third group is a *stilt gait* with a phantom; the patient experiences a phantom, but states that s/he has no illusion of using it. Walking with the prosthesis is experienced as walking with the stilt attached to the stump. The phantom leg may or may not follow the movements of the prosthetic knee joint. The fourth group has a *stilt gait without a phantom;* phantoms are absent, and the patients experience walking as with a stilt attached to the stump. Some patients can experience a clear phantom gait, even in cases with a markedly foreshortened phantom leg. If, however, the phantom location corresponds poorly with that of the prosthesis, it appears to be highly detrimental in the patient's ability to walk with a prosthesis. Foreshortening per se does not seem to matter. A marked discrepancy in phantom location is rare.

Crönholm (1951) points out that upper-limb amputees working with a prosthesis almost always have the experience of working with a tool attached to the stump whether or not they have a phantom sensation. He did have two cases in which patients had the experience of using the phantom hand when using the prosthesis. Crönholm asserts that, in some cases, if the prosthesis is hit, the patient experiences a sensation assigned to the phantom similar to that when a real limb is hit. Some patients feel they can twist their phantom ankle just like the real ankle if they make a false step with the prosthesis. If they walk in water, their phantom foot may feel wet. Some patients, when they have an itch in the phantom, automatically scratch the corresponding place on the prosthesis. While usually this does not influence the phantom itch, on occasion it does.

Crönholm (1951) discusses the reasons patients wear prostheses. He states that a leg amputee always wears a prosthesis in order to be able to walk. Its function is usually but not always purposive. It is usually constructed so that it moves very much the same way as a real leg. An arm amputee wears a prosthesis either to be able to perform certain functions or for cosmesis. Since the lower limb amputee uses his prosthesis in very much the same way as the normal leg, Crönholm says that it is easier for him to identify the phantom with a prosthesis. Since the upper-limb amputee uses his prosthesis in quite a different way from the real arm, the likelihood of identifying the phantom with a prosthesis is much less.

Bornstein (1949) says that interpretation of the phantom limb is linked with the psychic experience of body image. It is more likely to occur in persons in whom optic perceptions predominate over kinesthetic. Electroshock treatment was instituted in three cases. In all three, the phantom limb did not reappear for one and one-half years.

Weinstein et al. (1964) feel that their findings support the theory that the phantom limb has its origin in the sensory part of the cerebral cortex. They have demonstrated the existence of phantom sensation in cases of congenital aplasia. They feel that this suggests that the sensory homunculus is a sufficient condition for the production of a phantom. The incidence of phantom in congenital amelia is 18 percent. In older individuals, the incidence of phantoms in major limb amputation is between 90 to 100 percent. There were more phantoms in above-knee amputation as opposed to below-knee amputation. There was a higher incidence of phantom sensation when the hand or arm was lost as compared to only fingers being lost. Patients fitted with a prosthesis before the age of seven had a significantly higher incidence of phantom than those fitted later or not at all. Of the sixteen cases with congenital phantoms, 81.2 percent were fitted with a prosthesis before the age of seven, whereas of the seventy-eight cases who did not demonstrate congenital phantom, only 52.6 percent were fitted before the age of seven.

The onset of the phantom in congenital aplasia ranges from the time of earliest recollection (44%) to slightly prior to the time of the interview (28%). In only two cases had the phantom disappeared by the time of the interview. The quality of the phantom in congenital aplasia appeared as natural, whereas in acquired limb amputation most reports as to the quality can be categorized as painful, tingling, or natural.

Phantoms are varyingly reported as being consciously present during all waking hours or very infrequently. Patients with left lower-limb amputations experienced the phantom more frequently than did those with right lower-limb amputations. Those amputated before the age of four experienced a phantom less frequently. For congenital aplasia, it was surprising to me to find that 44 percent of those reporting phantoms felt the phantom at least daily. The parts perceived depended upon where the amputation was. Amputations above a joint caused more parts to be experienced. The side was also significant. Right below-elbow amputees felt more parts than left below-elbow amputees. For all groups, the more distal parts were more frequently felt. Strangely, while in the upper limb the above-joint amputees felt the distal parts more distinctly and felt more of them, for the lower limbs there was a complete reversal. Below-knee amputees tended to have a more complete phantom than above-knee amputees. Bilateral amputees were also examined. As with unilateral amputees, a greater number of parts were experienced on the left as opposed to the right. In congenital aplasias, 33 percent of the patients reported perception of their entire missing limb, but several reported feeling only an amorphous sensation extending but a few inches from the spine (22%). This phenomenon was not reported in any of the adult amputees. Of lower-limb amputees, 47 percent disliked the phantom sensation, while only 27 percent of arm amputees disliked it. Upper-limb amputees like the sensation in 13 percent of the cases and only 27 percent liked the feeling in leg amputees. The majority are indifferent to phantom sensation.

The tactual sensitivity of the amputation stump was significantly greater than the contralateral homologous area of the intact limb in the upper limb in two-point discrimination and point localization. In pressure sensitivity the difference was not significant.

The theories of phantom causation are (1) fantasy, (2) peripheral stimulation, and (3) central organization. The fantasy theory proposes that the phantom exists because the patient psychologically cannot accept the fact that he has lost a part. The phantom is the result of an individual's emotional need for that part. Weinstein (1968) found that there was no relationship between emotional significance and need and the occurrence of phantoms. This indicates that the emotional attitude towards the body part cannot predict the incidence of phantoms.

The peripheral theory attributes the phantom sensation to nervous activity in the stump provoked by various irritants. The central theory proposes that the neighboring cortical areas stimulate the cortical area representing the missing part. Weinstein (1968) avers that the data strongly support the theory that physiological factors are the main determinants of the phantom. He feels that the phantom originates in the sensory homunculus of the cerebral cortex.

Weinstein, Vetter, and Serson (1964) reiterate their findings of phantom limbs in five individuals with congenital aplasia and report thirteen additional cases. The percentage of congenital aplasia patients demonstrating phantoms is 18.3 percent. They point to the abolishment of the phantom sensation after excision of part of the postcentral gyrus in which the leg is represented. They also report that the incidence of phantom is higher in cases with terminal aplasia rather than intercalary aplasia. This is expected, since the representation of distal parts is greater than more proximal parts.

Phantoms acquired after amputation of congenitally deformed or aplastic parts was also reported. The phantoms were always those of the amputated parts and resembled the deformities, but never were an intact limb. My patients report the same. This finding is not consistent with the "wish-fulfillment" or "fantasy" theory.

In cases sustaining cerebral vascular accidents contralateral to the amputation, the phantom is abolished or diminished. Cerebral vascular accidents ipsilateral to the amputation cause no change in the phantom. A cerebral vascular accident prior to an amputation reduces the likelihood of a phantom, while the same accident after an amputation is associated with disappearance of a phantom. Central representation seems to be sufficient in Weinstein et al. (1964) view for the production of the phantom. They say that the experience can be modified by various means. Early environmental factors, such as stump or visual stimulation, may enhance the probability of eliciting a phantom in congenital limb-deficient children. Paraplegics have phantoms, as do patients with amputations of other body parts. It is proposed that phantoms of deafferented body parts are not telescoped as with amputees, because the visual experience of seeing the legs prevents perceptual distortion.

Good tactile sensitivity on the stump of amputees compared with the homologous areas on the intact limb was found by Weinstein et al. (1964). No such sensitivity difference between limbs was found by Wilson et al. (1962) in either of two nonamputee groups, one of which was blind. An unexpected finding was that there was greater sensitivity of even the intact limb of the amputee group. This suggested to the authors that the greatly reduced input affects the activity of both somatosensitive areas. The blind group also showed significantly lower thresholds than the sighted nonamputee group.

Haber (1955) says that even patients with a definite phantom sensation of the extremity never experience the feeling of having anything on the foot, such as a shoe or a bandage, even when they had such an object on the foot when the trauma occurred. I have had four cases of "phantom shoe," three cases of "phantom bandage," and one each of "phantom ring," and "phantom watch."

Pollock et al. (1957) say that the term *phantom limb* should be restricted to those instances in which a limb has been amputated. In injury to the spinal cord and cauda equina, three different types of sensation should be differentiated: proprioceptive and kinesthetic sensations; nociceptive or painful sensations; and awareness. They say that awareness of a limb is possible only when the lesion is incomplete or recovering. Recovery of deep sensibility is related to awareness more than are other modality sensations. When sensations are referred into insensate extremities, subsequent amputation does not result in any change. The sensation continues to be referred into the dismembered limb, as well as into the intact one.

Nociceptive and proprioceptive referred sensations are said to originate in the distal end of the proximal segment of the injured spinal cord. This is by no means certain. Sensory by-pass around a proved complete spinal cord lesion has been seen by this author in at least six cases.

When rhizotomy precedes an amputation, phantom limb does not develop. In all spinal cord injury patients, when nociceptive sensations were distally referred, they continued after rhizotomy. When proprioceptive sensations had been distally referred in one patient, they continued after rhizotomy. By anesthetizing the distal end of the proximal segment of the injured spinal cord, when one extremity has been amputated, nociceptive and proprioceptive distally referred sensations in the intact and absent extremities disappeared. Neither rhizotomy nor anesthetizing the distal segment of the spinal cord was effective.

Simmel (1956) reported that phantoms characteristically appear after amputation in patients with leprosy. They do not result from leprous absorption of digits, as long as surgery is not superimposed on the process of absorption. They appear when the remnants of partially absorbed digits are amputated, but they do not appear following plastic surgery of the hand long after absorption of the fingers is complete. The phantoms resulting from amputation of partially absorbed digits do not consist merely of the remnants that were surgically removed; they are phantoms of the whole digits prior to any absorption. Upon amputation of a leg, the toes of which had been absorbed prior to the amputation, the phantom experience is complete, including the toes. Simmel's (1956) conclusion is that the following variables do *not* influence the appearance of the phantom:

(A) Age at the time of loss, provided amputations in early childhood are excluded.

(B) The time elapsed since amputation.

(C) The nature of the condition which makes amputation necessary.
(D) The delay between the original injury or infection and the time of amputation.
(E) The presence of pain prior to or following amputation.

The basic phantom phenomenon is postulated by Kolb (1954) to be the function of the sensory motor cortex. A second type of stump sensation is stronger; momentary paresthetic "pins and needles" sensations occur by touching neuromas in the stump. This is dependent upon functional activity of lower spinal centers. In addition, there are stump pains brought on by prosthetic socket irritation, injury or disease of the limb remnant, etc., some of which may be referred distally. Stump pain is not to be confused with phantom pain.

Chapter VIII

# PHANTOM PAIN AND ITS TREATMENT

In addition to Chapter VII's phantom sensation, there is a phenomenon termed *phantom pain,* which is quite different and by definition disagreeable. It may vary from a paresthesia type of pain, which varies from "pins and needles" to an electric-shock-like phenomenon, usually but not always elicited by pressure over a neuroma. It may have a burning and agonizingly painful nature. Another type of painful phantom is a cramping sensation in the part. This is usually quite unpleasant. In cases where amputation is not possible immediately after severe crush injury or other types of trauma, phantom pain is quite common and may be agonizing. Phantom pain frequently persists indefinitely.

Bilateral amputations may be followed by bi- or unilateral phantom hands or feet. One may be painful and one painless. Intractable pain in the phantom, while rare, may present a formidable therapeutic problem. It generally appears about the same time as the phantom, immediately or some time after the operation and is felt mainly in the hand or foot. In the hand, pain is referred chiefly to the wrist, palm, knuckles, and tips of the fingers and thumb. In the foot the insteps, heels, and toes are felt most. If there was a painful wound prior to the amputation, the pain may persist in the same area.

The sensations experienced in the phantom are those of warmth, numbness, smarting, shooting, compression, itching, burning, heaviness, throbbing, piercing, cramping, sticking, or cutting. It is usually continuous and subject to exacerbations. There may be a sensation of the phantom limb being crushed or torn (Editorial, *JAMA*, 1944). The supposition that the condition is psychogenic has not been borne out by clinical observations. Electrical stimulation of the brachial plexus long after amputation reproduced the sensation of a hand that was bent and hurt. The worst painful phantoms are cases of interstitial neuritis or abnormally large and tender neuromas. In these cases, any stimulus, physical or emotional, that can evoke pain is usually effective both for stump and phantom limb. Then, cramplike rigidity of the phantom hand and fingers usually forms the most constant background of pain. Pain in the phantom may be due to excessive stimulation of the nerves in the stump and results in painful representation of the absent limb in the phantom and limits voluntary movement of the phantom only because voluntary efforts aggravate the pain. The prevailing posture of the phantom is that of the part at the time of the amputation.

Dessaint (Rouen) studied 1000 cases of amputees and noted a striking parallel between painful rhythms of stump pain and the course of gastric ulcers. He said that the pain appeared at fixed hours and it seems to be due to difficulty with chemical transmission of the nerve impulse.

Fontaine et al. of Strasbourg (1949) observed 586 cases. Of the amputees, 82 percent had more or less phantom sensation but only 6 percent had really painful stumps, 12 percent of which were from civil practice, 6 percent from World War I, and 4 percent from World War II. Pain is more frequent in amputations due to trauma (14%) than those to arterial disease (6%). They state that sympathetic nervous intervention and resection of a bad scar is better than intervention on a spinal cord or nerve root, since the latter has given only poor results. They also recommend direct cerebral intervention.

The intensity of phantom pain varies in different individuals and from time to time. The patient's attitude toward amputation and to his social position is particularly important, as is his basic pain tolerance. The abnormal sensations at times assigned to the phantom pain are very intense in some cases and very unpleasant. In about one third of the cases, the abnormal sensations are less pronounced, although still painful. In the third group, the abnormal sensations have merely insignificant intensity. This includes almost one half of the cases. Those cases with abnormal sensations are primarily in cases with continuous basic phantom sensation; where the basic phantom is intermittent, only a few patients have severe phantom pain. Some cases reported as having "phantoms" are not true phantom sensation, but are a part of the stump percept. Crönholm (1951) states that his was not a random sample, since arm amputees predominated. Many of the cases were seen because they were complaining of pain.

High-intensity abnormal sensations (pain) are experienced more frequently by distal than by proximal amputees, but there is no difference in the upper and lower limb. Older amputees have more severe pain, which is usually experienced a short time after amputation. The phantom may change in severity and quality after operations performed for pain relief.

Crönholm points out that the pain may be linked to the way the patient has experienced the limb before amputation. Affective factors are of very great importance in the way the patient experiences the phantom pain which may explain part of the severity soon after limb ablation.

Browder and Gallagher (1946) report that none of their seven congenital limb-deficient amputees had ever been aware of a phantom limb. Of the remaining ninety-three amputees, seventy-nine admitted phantom sensation. Ten patients had enduring painful phantoms with pain of abnormal posture. This group of patients appeared to have two distinct types of discomfort The first and most outstanding one is the unalterable, often distorted posture assumed by the phantom which results in a cramplike pain, mostly in the distal part of the phantom. The amputated member is said to feel as if it were clenched in a vise in this fixed position. The digits are frequently described as "dug into" the palm or sole. The second is the shocklike sensation, or cutting.

Foerster (1931) says that the person not only feels the limb is still connected with the body, but has certain definite sensations. He states that the hand or the fingers are generally warmer than the remaining hand. Rarely do they feel cold. The pains are characterized as piercing, cutting, or burning. Some feel them constantly and others only periodically. Many have the sensation of crushing. The pains may be so severe that many of these persons become addicted to narcotics. Attempts to influence the pain by suggestion were found useless. One patient who had the feeling that his thumb was piercing his hand, would overcome this pain by volition, i.e. when he made a mental effort to pull the thumb out of his hand, the pain disappeared. The pain reappeared when he discontinued this act. A number of persons state that the phantom limb feels shorter and more slender than the healthy one, and that it becomes gradually shorter in the course of time. Amputated painful hands and legs are generally in abnormal positions.

The cramping type of pain is usually associated with a vivid picture of the position of the amputated extremity. Usually, these patients describe the position of the amputated extremity in great detail. They feel that motion of the part alleviates the pain. This, in fact, is frequently the case. If the normal extremity is placed in the cramped position and the patient is instructed to do exercises both with the normal extremity and with the phantom extremity, motion of the stump muscles is usually observed. If this is repeated often enough, this type of phantom pain disappears, in many cases.

Prolonged phantom pain does not spontaneously abate or disappear. This pain does not change in severity from week to week, whereas those in whom the pain is destined to disappear spontaneously usually show more or less progressive diminution of pain within two weeks following amputation.

At the end of one month, two thirds of patients with transitory painful phantoms are pain-free, although they do have a phantom sensation, which, in some cases, persists intermittently for years.

Dederich (1970) discusses pain after amputation. Few patients who have had amputations do not experience the pain that in Germany is commonly called *nerve pain*. It usually disappears rapidly. The pain occurs either in the stump or in the missing part of the limb or alternates between each, but rarely in both simultaneously. It is difficult to locate or measure and appears to affect different subjects with different intensity.

Burning pain is the very center of the thoughts and lives of many patients who have had amputations. They crave pain-free stumps, pain-free sleep, and the ability to do their work free of pain. Dederich avers that some patients have undergone as many as thirty-five operations for the treatment of burning pain alone and that many seek relief with alcohol or drugs. Myoplastic surgical revision of the stumps has helped many of these unfortunates, according to Dederich.

The second type of pain, usually transient, is sharp and lancinating. Usually, this is superimposed upon a painless phantom sensation or upon any of the other types of phantom pain. This usually seems to have its origin in the stump and, most commonly, is due to pressure over a neuroma from the socket of a prosthesis, or the neuroma may be pressed upon by muscular contractions. Adhesions between the neuroma and the underlying tissues may cause traction on the neuroma. This type of pain may come from any type of pressure over the nerve.

The most common type of stump neuralgia is that associated with excessive mesoblastic and axonal growth at the end of a larger peripheral nerve. This type of pain is electriclike and shooting. It is often initiated by pressure or other mechanical stimuli. In some cases, it is associated with a "jumping stump." The pain of a stump neuralgia is intermittent, sharp, and shooting in character. It arises in the stump and radiates into the phantom rather than residing in it. This pain is apparently due to a neuroma. Stump neuralgias are best treated by resection of the neuroma and revision of the stump.

It is often very difficult for the patient to differentiate between pain in the stump and abnormal sensation, such as dysesthesias, paresthesias, "nerve vibrations," "electric shock," and "numbness."

Some part of phantom-limb sensation and/or pain may vanish after resection of neuromas, but this is often not the case. Anesthesia of the stump may cause disappearance of phantom in some cases. Spinal anesthesia need not cause the phantom to vanish. Even operations on the peripheral nerves, the dorsal spinal roots and the spinal cord including anterolateral cordotomy, posterior cordotomy, etc., need not always cause disappearance of the phantom.

The "temperature" of the phantom may be influenced by whether the stump is hot or cold. Sometimes a phantom can be restimulated after disappearance by faradic electrical stimulation of the stump. Operations on the sympathetic nervous system may alleviate the pains of amputees, but not in all cases. Frontal lobotomy often causes the phantom pain to become less clear and experienced less frequently, but it may also continue as before. After cerebral vascular accidents or after resection of a part of the parietal cortex, contralateral to the amputation, there may or may not be disappearance of the phantom sensation and/or pain. A number of unknown factors appear to be concerned, both peripheral and central, making therapeutic efforts difficult.

Herrmann and Gibbs (1945) do not believe that the symptoms are purely psychic, but they feel that peripheral irritation, while by no means constituting the whole story, does represent an important factor in the syndrome of phantom-limb pain. The authors ligated the large nerves with nonabsorbable material without preliminary crush of the nerve. Of the 121 patients who could be followed, 113 stated that they had never experienced phantom limb pain after the operation. Only 5.8 percent of the group complained of phantom limb pain. All but one of the patients who complained of phantom limb pain were in the sixth or seventh decades of life. All were male and had gangrene due to arterial insufficiency or arterial thrombosis.

Herrmann and Gibbs (1945) recommend placing a tight ligature about the uninjured large nerve trunk at a point about 1 inch above the level of amputation. This they regard as a simple and physiologic method of preventing regeneration of axons from the cut end of the nerve. The incidence of phantom limb pain in the series of 120 patients was highest (25%) for the 4 patients with severely traumatized limbs, but was only 5.8 percent for the entire group. The distinction between phantom-limb sensation and phantom pain was not adequately differentiated in their paper, in my opinion. Furthermore, their incidence of phantom sensation and pain is identical to those of others using different treatment (Fontaine et al., 1949).

White (1943) states that if there is a painful neuroma, excision of the neuroma is worth *one* surgical trial if done early, provided the pain disappears when the neuroma is injected with procaine. Repeated excisions, neurectomies, reamputations, and resection of posterior roots consistently fail. White (1944) also states that neurectomy by injection or by section is always unsuccessful. Reamputation for pain alone is useless. It may be useful in conjunction with a refashioning of the stump for other purposes, such as scar resection. Stump pain may be caused by a neuroma, poorly fitting socket, tumor, or injury.

The burning pain is thought to have a neurovascular component and to be similar to causalgia. It may be related to interstitial neuritis. This pain is the most unremitting and devastating type of pain. It is a frequent cause for suicide in the amputee. It is agonizing in nature, and attempts at relief have been remarkably ineffective. Sympathetic blocks, sympathectomies, as well as progressive sectioning of the pain and sympathetic pathways, have been attempted with little success. Cold saline spinal washes and electrical stimulation, both central and peripheral, have not as yet proved their worth, despite early enthusiasm.

When spinal segments are stimulated that refer pain to a part of an absent limb, a foreshortened, painless phantom tends to grow to its normal length. There is usually severe pain in the phantom in the location served by the spinal segment, which frequently is followed by numbness of the phantom and the pain. The parts of the phantom that previously were absent often tend to fill in and to remain complete for some time. On occasion, an area of painful phantom disappears after stimulation of its radicular segment by hypertonic saline or other chemical agents. The effect of the injection of various solutions, such as local anesthetics or hypertonic saline, into various spinal segments is variable. They seem to alter the central excitatory state of the central nervous system in some obscure fashion and, thereby, change the phantom sensation and/or pain. In patients having complaints of pain in the stump and phantom during ejaculation, defecation, and urination, this usually diminishes with time and has been speculated to be due to postoperative congestion in the pelvis (Slocum, 1949). Patients should be reassured that it rarely lasts more than for a six-month period and usually disappears spontaneously.

Stump pain and referred pain, causalgias, and neuralgias must be differentiated from true, painful phantom. Causalgia infrequently follows major amputations. It is diagnosed by a cold, clammy, sweaty and cyanotic hand, foot, or stump associated with a burning type of pain. It may occur after a minor amputation. The stump and surrounding area are exquisitely sensitive. The slightest superficial touch or temperature change may precipitate an explosive, burning pain that radiates up the extremity and lasts long after the stimulus has been withdrawn. A phantom part may be present, but the causalgic pain is not usually referred to the absent part. Causalgias are sometimes relieved by either surgical or chemical interruption of the sympathetic pathways serving the affected part. Large doses of anticholinergic drugs are helpful to many of my patients. Biofeedback has helped a few cases, as has electrical nerve stimulation.

White (1944) states that in a stump with distal pain, which is cold, clammy, and cyanotic, sympathectomy may be a very effective treatment.

Sympathetic blocking should be done first, since this is frequently successful and may permanently relieve the pain. Repeated blocks may be done if the pain relief persists.

Repeated injections of sympathetic ganglia produce, in some cases of burning phantom limb, beneficial effects that persist for weeks or months. The beneficial effects from this therapy are only temporary (Leriche, 1937, 1939, 1939).

If pain relief occurs with each block, but the period of relief is short, then sympathectomy is indicated. If an effective block occurs with absence of sweating and the pain is not relieved, then sympathectomy will be unsuccessful and should not be performed. White (1944) says that posterior rhizotomy and intrathecal alcohol are ineffective. He asserts that spinothalamic tractotomy is good, provided the pain in the stump is confined to the stump alone. White alleges that a disagreeable phantom sensation is not relieved, even by cordotomy.

While the results of these measures are at times only transitory, they are the best procedures available. Anterolateral cordotomy is necessary only in unusual instances. Lasting, painful phantom often elicits many attempts at treatment, e.g. revisional reamputation of the stump, excision of stump neuromas, division of nerve trunks at higher levels, various types of injections aimed to interrupt the peripheral nerves of the stump, dorsal root rhizotomy, anterolateral cordotomy, paravertebral alcohol injections, sympathetic ganglionectomy, and prefrontal lobotomy. Browder and Gallagher (1946) say they have been "guilty" of trying all of these singly and in combination in attempts to relieve the pain of the painful phantom, but they now believe they should be separately and collectively condemned as therapeutic measures for this disorder. They say the only probable method for relief of enduring painful phantom limb is interruption of proprioceptive sensibility of the involved part. This can be accomplished either by section of a dorsal column of the spinal cord or by excision of a part of the parietal cortex. These procedures should be carried out only in patients with complaints of intractable pain, resulting from abnormal posture of the phantom limb. Their experience indicates that dorsal cordotomy seemingly abolishes the patient's knowledge of the posture of a phantom foot and concomitantly the cramplike pain associated with the distorted posture. It should therefore be used mainly for the cramplike pain, and not the other types.

Falconer and Lindsay (1946) report two cases of painful phantom in the upper limb, relieved by high cervical cordotomy performed by controlled graduated division under local anesthesia. They say there is a group of patients who get relief from interruption of peripheral or sympathetic nerve pathways, in whom pain impulses appear to arise in or around the neuromas of divided nerves. The two reported individuals belong to the other main group, in which painful impulses arise in the dorsal horn cells of the spinal cord. They declare they can be relieved only by section of the spinothalamic tract or by excision of the sensory cortex of the cerebrum. They say that infiltration of the appropriate peripheral or sympathetic pathways with a local anesthetic is useful diagnostically to distinguish between the two groups. When infiltration fails to give relief, section of the spinothalamic tract is suggested and seems preferable to ablation of the sensory cortex, because it does not destroy postural and other discriminative sensations in the stump, but only abstracts from it the sensation of pain. The stump is still functionally useful.

In some cases of phantom pain, nerve block with alcohol or phenol to destroy the nerve tracts may occasionally be successful. In other cases, some patients have phantom and/or stump pain relieved by the constriction of a prosthetic socket. In these cases, the pain may be relieved by total contact casts left on and changed weekly. When a prosthesis is again used, the patient usually is free of pain. Sometimes, a hard plastic laminate socket, total contact in design and held on by elastic strapping, needs to be used whenever the prosthesis is not worn. The etiology of this type of pain is not understood, but may be related to sensory deprivation.

James Campbell (1972), who has done much work on control of phantom pain, says that for the upper limb, his experience indicates that rhizotomy, sympathectomy, and the capping of nerve ends with Millipore® porous plastic or silicone rubber are not successful in controlling phantom pain.

Kolb (1954) reports one case who had undergone twenty-seven surgical and anesthetic procedures in thirty years, including resection of the somatosensory cortex without modification of his painful phantom. Kolb recommends proper preparation of the patient about to undergo an amputation. He says this may prevent the development of the painful phantom limb "hallucination." It should include a discussion of the occurrence of the phantom limb phenomenon and an inquiry into the patient's desires and fears in regard to the disposal of the part to be amputated.

Arthur Battista (1972) is attempting to reduce the severity and incidence of painful phantoms by three experimental procedures. The first is the wash of the spinal cord by cold saline. The second is the use of stimulation over the peripheral nerve by an implanted stimulator. When the patient has discomfort, he stimulates his own nerve, thereby decreasing its potential for excitation. The third technique is stimulation of the nerve, but at the level of the posterior columns that convey sensation rather than over the peripheral nerve. Each of the three techniques is experimental and significant series of cases are as yet not available. A number of failures using these methods are known to me.

Neuralgias of the stump are classified into two categories. One is a more or less continuous, dull ache usually near the end of a major amputation stump, somewhat aggravated by pressure, said to be more severe in damp weather. This presents a formidable problem in prosthetic fitting. It is due to some pathologic alteration in the cut ends of the bone and muscles and thus is a category of stump, rather than phantom, pain. The second type of pain is a deep-seated, burning and boring type of discomfort usually in the distal part of the phantom. Patients who have been designated as having transitory painful phantoms describe only the deep-seated burning and boring pain.

For diagnostic purposes, if a local anesthetic is injected into the nerve, this may provide relief if the cause of the pain is distal. While many prefer to inject the area of maximum tenderness locally, my experience has been that if the nerve is injected proximal to the point of maximal tenderness the information gained is more reliable. Thus, if I suspect a neuroma is the cause of pain in the below-knee stump, I inject the appropriate nerve proximal to the knee. In this way, the peripheral causes will not be able to transmit their impulses to the central nervous system. This method of evaluation has the advantage that it helps differentiate those causes of phantom pain in the peripheral nerves but proximal to the stump, such as the referred pain from a herniated intervertebral disk on the amputated side Local injections, frequently with an anesthetic and steroid anti-inflammatory agent, are sometimes helpful in the treatment, as well as the evaluation of phantom pain. In this case, injection at the point of maximal tenderness is used.

Amputees are not immune to other diseases and illnesses. The pain felt at the lateral border of the foot in herniation of an intervertebral disk may be exactly the same in an amputee, even when the leg is absent. Radiation of pain from a central location is felt as if the limb were present. Spinal cord tumors and diseases of internal organs or stimulation of the brain refer the pain to the amputated extremity.

Another type of pain is described as twisting, burning, pulling, or itching. This symptom is usually intermittent and is more gnawing than agonizing. It may be brought on by stimulation of the stump, urination in the lower-limb amputee, weather changes, and emotionally charged events.

Finneson et al. (1957) report two cases of radicular pain caused by a herniated nucleus pulposus and phantom limb symptoms existing simultaneously in the same extremity. The independence of each modality was demonstrated by postoperative disappearance of the radicular pain with persistence of phantom limb symptoms. The following factors aid in arriving at the diagnosis of herniated nucleus pulposus in the presence of an ipsilateral amputation:

1. The history of a change in the pattern of the phantom-limb symptoms, as well as the appearance of low-back symptoms and signs.
2. The radicular component of pain is referred to the phantom limb as if projected to the normal dermatome distribution of a specific lumbar or cervical nerve root.
3. The straight leg raising test (as executed with the amputation stump) is positive when the amputation is below the knee, but absent when the amputation is above the knee.
4. Electromyography and nerve conduction studies are abnormal.
5. Myelography confirms the presumptive clinical diagnosis.

Painful phantom should be differentiated from other causes of pain in the stump, such as pain in a scar, usually due to a nerve bound down into the scar, adherent scars, referred pain, bursitis over a spur, or neuroma. For these other causes of pain, conservative treatment should be used first. Operative measures have been rarely successful. Conservative therapy includes wearing the artificial limb and a night plaster-of-paris socket, elastic bandaging night and day, ultrasound therapy over the nerve trunk and neuroma, percussion therapy for desensitization, negative galvanism, paraffin baths, and diathermy. I have found these to be of benefit in some cases. If the above are not successful, the injection of local anesthetic, with or without cortisone, may be of help. In my experience, the use of a suspension of cortisone is inadvisable, since it tends to cause scarring. I prefer the clear solutions of cortisone or cortisonelike compounds These are much less irritating than the crystalline suspensions both acutely and over a long-term period.

Percussion should be general and localized to the neuroma. In this technique, a small-diameter rod is placed over the most tender part of the neuroma, and a mallet is used by the patient to strike the rod, which in turn transmits the force to the neuroma. This is extremely painful so the patient must control the intensity. It should be done many times a day. Usually with time the patient can tolerate more percussion as the nerve scars down due to the repeated injury. In cases of extreme tenderness, a sphygmomanometer or a tourniquet can be placed above the neuroma. When this is used, a relative anoxia of the nerve occurs, making the neuroma less sensitive, thus allowing tapping with less pain. While this technique is effective, I have found that it is rarely necessary.

All of the complaints referred to a stump are not necessarily due either to local conditions in the stump nor to the use of a prosthesis. Systemic diseases may be causing the symptoms. Psychological diseases may manifest themselves by somatization. There are hysterical manifestations in certain amputees. These may manifest themselves by unusual complaints of local pain, phantom pain, or sensitivity to the prosthesis. Classical hysteria may occur with hysterical joint flexion, which may lead to organic flexion contractures.

## Neurologic Stump Changes

Neuromas are always formed when a nerve is cut. After amputation, stumps frequently have hyperactivity in the stump musculature. Fascicular twitchings of small muscle bundles often appear. At times, there is spasmodic jerking of the stump. It is involuntary. In some patients, the stump has periods of sustained clonic contractions. They may be caused by passive or active movement of the stump or other parts of the body, various stimuli, such as sudden sounds, urination, defecation, or orgasm, strong and sudden light, and occasionally by psychogenic factors. Increased deep tendon reflexes in the stump and neighboring parts of the body have been recorded. There seems to be hyperactivity of the autonomic nervous system, as evidenced by vasomotor disturbances and hyperhidrosis. There is an occasional patient with increased pilomotor activity.

About one half of the patients in Crönholm's study (1951) had spontaneous muscular hyperactivity in the stump. The intensity and frequency of this activity vary considerably. In more than one half of the amputees, there is hyperactivity of the deep tendon reflexes. The activity in the stump can sometimes be increased by stimulating the stump. There may be abnormal sensation both at the stimulated area and the referred area, or sensations with abnormal localization with pain, but with a normally localized sensation which is not painful. Three basic theories have been given for these phenomena: (1) If the same sensory nerve has fibers with branches to the inner organs and the skin, this may cause them. (2) A spinal mechanism may be responsible in that the afferents from viscera and cutaneous regions, both end on the same spinothalamic tract neurons. (3) The referred pain is caused by cerebral summation of impulses from the viscera and the skin, and localization is determined by the cortical integration of these impulses through central spread of excitation.

Both hyposensitivity and hypersensitivity to various kinds of stimuli are often present in the stump, on the trunk, either generally or segmentally, or at distal sites, such as parts of the face. This seems to be a phenomenon similar to peripheral neuropathy.

# BIBLIOGRAPHY


Barker, R. G., Wright, B. A., Myerson, L., and Gonick, M. R.: Adjustment to Physical Handicap and Illness—A Survey of the Social Psychology of Physique and Disability, 2nd ed. *NY Soc Sci Res Coun, Bull* No. 55, 1953.

Battista, A.: Experiments on reducing phantom pain. Personal communication with the author, 1972.

Berger, N.: Studies of the upper extremity amputee. *Artif Limbs, 5:*57-72, 1958.

Bornstein, P. A.: Phenomenon of the phantom limb. *Encephale, 38:*1-48, 1949.

Browder, J. and Gallagher, J. F.: Surgical treatment of painful phantom limb. *NY State J Med, 46, 21:*2403-2405, 1946.

Brown, P. W.: Bilateral lower extremity amputee. *J Bone Joint Surg, 52A, 4:*687-700, 1970.

Burgess, E. M., Romano, R. L., Zettl, J. H., and Schrock, R. D. Jr.: Amputations of the leg for peripheral vascular insufficiency. *J Bone Joint Surg, 53A, 5:*874-890, 1971.

Campbell, J.: Personal communication with the author.

Crönholm, B.: Phantom Limbs in Amputees. *Journal Acta Psychiatrica et Neurologica Suppl, 72,* 1951.

Dederich, R.: *Amputationen der Unteren Extraemitaeten.* Stuttgart, Georg Thieme Verlag, 1970.

Dederich, R.: *Amputationen der Unteren Extraemitaten,* Georg Thieme Verlag, Stuttgart, 1970.

Falconer, M. A. and Lindsay, J. S. B.: Painful Phantom Limb Treated by High Cervical Cordotomy: Report of Two Cases. *Br J Surg, 33:*301-306, April, 1946.

Finneson, B. E., Haft, H., and Krueger, E. G.: Phantom limb syndrome associated with herniated nucleus pulposis. *J Neurol, 14, 3:*344-346, 1957.

Fishman, S.: Amputee needs, frustrations and behavior. *Rehabil Lit, 20, 11:*322-329, 1959.

Fishman, S.: In Garrett, J. F. and Levine, E. S.: *Psychological Practices with the Physically Handicapped.* New York, Columbia U Pr, 1962.

Foerster, O.: Phantom limb. *Med Klin Berlin, 27:*497-500, 1931.

Fontaine, R., Frank, P., and Chorwath, V.: Contribution a L'Etude des

Gangrenes Limitees des Orteils avec Conservation du Pouls et des Oscillations. *Arch Mal Coeur 42:*240-245, Feb., 1949.

Friedmann, L. W.: Amputations and prostheses in primitive cultures. *Bull Prosthet Res, 10, 17:*105-138, 1972.

Friedmann, L. W., Katz, J. F., and Siffert, R. S.: *Skeletal Attachment and Transcutaneous Passage of Upper Extremity Prostheses—A Review and Preliminary Report.* Proceedings of the Twelfth Congress of the International Society of Orthopedic Surgery and Traumatology, Tel Aviv, Oct. 9-12, 1972. International Congress Series No. 291, Amsterdam, Excerpta Medica.

Gillis, L.: *Artificial Limb.* London, Pitman Med. Publ. Ltd., 1957.

Harber, W. B.: Effects of loss of limb on sensory functions. *J Psychol, 40:* 115-123, 1955.

———: Observations of phantom limb phenomena. *AMA Arch Neurol Psychiatry, 75:*624-636, 1956.

Haj, F.: *Disability in Antiquity.* New York, Philos Lib, 1970.

Henderson, and Smyth:

Herrmann, L. G. and Gibbs, E. W.: Phantom limb pain. *Am J Surg, 47, 2:*24-36, 1945.

Höllander, E.: Die chirurgische saege. *Arch Klin Chir, 106:*317-336, 1915.

Holling, H. E.: *Peripheral Vascular Diseases.* Philadelphia, Lippincott, 1972.

*JAMA,* Editorial, *125:*634, July 1, 1944.

Kallio, E. E.: Phantom limb of forearm stump cleft by kineplastic surgery. *J Int Chir, 12:*110-119, 1952.

Kessler, H. H.: Psychological preparation of the amputee. *Ind Med Surg, 20:*3, 1951.

Kinnier-Wilson, A. B.: Specifications of a loss. In Murdoch, G.: *Prosthetic and Orthotic Practice.* London, Edward Arnold Publishers, 1970, pp. 356-362.

Knapp, M. E.: Lower extremity amputations and prosthetics. *Postgrad Med, 44, 5:*259-264, 1968.

Kolb, L. C.: *The Painful Phantom—Psychology, Physiology, Treatment.* Springfield, Thomas, 1954.

Leriche, R.: A propos de 13 cas de desarticulation de la nanche. *Mem Acad de Chir, 63:*1435-1438, Dec. 22, 1937.

———: Moignons utiles et moignons inutilisables du membre inferieur; de la necesite d'une connaissance exacte des exigences de la prothèse dans la choix du niveau de l'amputation. *Presse Med, 47:*1333-1334, Sept. 13, 1939.

———: Moignons utiles et moignons inutilisables de la valeur compares des diverses amputations et desarticulations du membre superiour. *Presse Med, 47:*1350, Sept., 1939.

Livingston, K. E.: Phantom limb syndrome. *J Neurosurg,* May, 1945.

McKenzie, D. S.: Congenital deficiencies of the lower limb. In Murdoch, G.: *Prosthetic and Orthotic Practice.* London, Edward Arnold Publishers, 1970, pp. 315-327.

———: Functional replacement of the upper extremity today. In Murdoch, G.: *Prosthetic and Orthotic Practice.* London, Edward Arnold Publishers, 1970, pp. 363-376.

Marquardt, E. G.: *The Total Treatment of the Limb-deficient Child.* Rehabilitation Monograph No. 44, Institute of Rehabilitation Medicine, New York University Medical Center, 1969.

Mitchell, S. W.: *Injuries to Nerves and Their Consequences,* 1872.

Paré, A.: *Dix Livres de la Chirurgie.* Paris, 1564.

*Penthouse:* Forum: Art and amputees. *Penthouse, 3, 10:*14-18, June, 1972.

———: Forum: Art and amputees. *Penthouse, 4, 1:*133, Sept., 1972.

———: Forum: Art and amputees. *Penthouse, 4, 5:*17-21, Jan., 1973.

———: Forum: Art and amputees. *Penthouse, 4, 6:*14-16, Feb., 1973.

———: Forum: Art and amputees. *Penthouse, 4, 8:*16, Apr., 1973.

———: Forum: Art and amputees. *Penthouse, 4, 10:*24-26, June, 1973.

———: Forum: Art and amputees. *Penthouse, 4, 13:*128, Sept., 1973.

———: Forum: Monopede mania. *Penthouse, 4, 4:*12, Dec., 1972.

———: Forum: Monopede mania. *Penthouse, 4, 7:*18-20, Mar., 1973.

———: Forum: Monopede mania. *Penthouse, 4, 9:*24, May, 1973.

———: Forum: More monopede mania. *Penthouse, 4, 12:*20-30, Aug., 1973.

———: Forum: Special preference. *Penthouse, 4, 11:*20-26, July, 1973.

Pitres, Albert; and Vaillard (1887) in "A History of Medicine" by Fielding H. Garrison, 4th Ed. W. B. Saunders, Phila., 1929, reprinted 1966.

Pollock, L. J., Boshis, B., Arieff, A. J., Finkelman, I., Brown, M., Dobin, N. B., Kessert, B., Pyzik, S., Finkle, J. R., Tigay, E., and Zivin, I.: Phantom limb in patients with injuries to the spinal cord and cauda equina. *Surg Gynecol Obstet, 104:*407-415, 1957.

Resnik, H. L. D.: Suicide attempt by a ten-year-old after a quadruple amputation. *JAMA, 202, 7:*1011-1012, 1970.

Shaples, G. P.: *Ned: Child Amputee: Disabilities and Outcomes.* 1969.

Siller, J. and Silverman, S.: Studies of upper extremity amputees—Psychological factors. *Artif Limbs,* :88-116, 1958.

Simmel, M. L.: Phantoms in patients with leprosy and in elderly digital amputees. *Am J Psychol, 69, 4:*529-545, 1956.

Simpson, E. B.: *Individual Variations and Psychological Reaction to Amputation.* Biomechanics Laboratory, University of California at San Francisco-Berkeley. Publ. No. 35, 1959.

Slocum, D. B.: *An Atlas of Amputations.* St. Louis, Mosby, 1949.

Strudwick, P.: Up the shining mountain. *Runner's World, 7, 6:*30-33, 1972.

Stud with a stump. *Screw, 410:*4-7, 1977.

Syme, J.: *Principles of Surgery,* 3rd ed. London, H. Bealliere, 1942.

*The Star:* Ghost limbs by a one-armed man. *The Star,* Oct. 27, 1924.

Thorp, R.: *Slaves.* New York, M. Evans, 1972.

Warren, R. and Record, E. E.: *Lower Extremity Amputation for Arterial Insufficiency.* Boston, Little, 1967.

Weinstein, S.: The phantom experience. In Wright, G. N. and Beck-Trotter, A.: *Rehabilitation Research.* Madison, U of Wis Pr, 1968.

Weinstein, S., Vetter, R. J., and Serson, E. A.: *Physiological and Experiential Concomitants of the Phantom.* Vocational Rehabilitation Administration Grant No. 427, June, 1959-May, 1964.

Weiss, M., Gawronski, R., Gielsynski, A., Groski, W., Fituko, R., Kowalski M., Paradystal, R., Makowski, J., and Wirski, J.: *Myoplastic Amputation, Immediate Prosthesis and Early Ambulation.* Washington, D.C., Department of Health, Education and Welfare, Public Health Service, and National Institutes of Health, 1971.

White, J. C.: Causalgia and amputation stump pain. In: *Lectures on Peace and War Orthopedic Surgery.* Ann Arbor, Edwards Bros, 1943, pp. 80-83.

———: Pain after amputation and its treatment. *JAMA, 124:*1030, 1944.

White, Wright, and Dembo: Studies in adjustment to visible injuries: Evaluation of curiosity by the injured. *J Abnorm Psychol, 43:*18-28, 1948.

Wilson, A. B. Jr.: Some observations on upper extremity prosthetics. In Murdoch, G.: *Prosthetic and Orthotic Practice.* London, Edward Arnold Publishers, 1970.

Wilson, J. J., Wilson, B. C., and Swinyard, C. A.: Two point discrimination in congenital amputees. *J Comp Physiol Psychol, 55, 4:*482-485, 1962.

Wolff, P.: Footloose and fancy free. *Cheri, 1, 7:*43-92, 1977.

Wright, B. A.: *Psychology and Rehabilitation.* Washington, D.C., Am Psychol, 1959.

Wright, B. A.: *Physical Disability: A Psychological Approach.* New York, Harper Bros, 1960.

# INDEX

## D

## K



## L



## M



## N

## O



## P